Becoming the New You: The You You Want to Be

Michael Schwartz, N.D.

Becoming the New You: The You You Want to Be
Copyright © 2022 Michael Schwartz

Published by Center for Universal Teachings Applied
6003 Randolph Blvd
San Antonio, TX 78233

Scripture quotations are taken from the King James Version. Public domain.

ISBN: 979-8-9868249-2-5
eBook ISBN: 79-8-9868249-3-2
Cover design by rosecreativemarketing@gmail.com

Library of Congress Cataloguing-in-Publication Data:

Printed in the United States of America

—Objectivity

—Honesty

—Healing

—Love

Preface

The book you've chosen contains the methods and techniques for improving your life on multiple levels. Guaranteed! Of course, you must first become proficient in the concepts presented, then integrate and apply the methods and techniques daily. This process requires a commitment and a willingness to see life from a new perspective. But from personal experience, I can verify that the time and energy you put into your personal development is worth it.

The following material will reveal the complex workings of the human mind. More specifically, I will explain how the mind draws upon concepts housed and maintained in the subconscious mind. Concepts are the building blocks of thought, which then get categorized into language, ideas, images, and memories. Concepts intersect with one another to form the foundation of who you believe you should be and how you believe you should act and respond in every situation. Additionally, I will examine the behavioral patterns that enforce and validate those beliefs established by the subconscious concepts. Finally, I will present transformational methods and techniques for you to gain control over your negative behavioral patterns and cultivate balance within your whole being.

The ultimate goal of this work is to assist you in becoming the person you want to be. One who enjoys peace, balance, harmony, and excellent health on all levels.

Introduction

The following information presented on these pages will change your life, if applied. Why do I confidently believe this book is like a transformational key? Because when placed in the proper hands, the hands of one led by intuition and instinct to stop what they are doing and disrupt their mental and behavioral status quo, it will feel like unlocking a new level of their soul. A level that provides clarity, peace, divine love, divine guidance, and wisdom, to name a few benefits.

I can verify these methods because I've been in the role of student (seeker) and went through this process from the ground level. The teachings within this book felt like divine downloads—as well as a call to action! I was tasked with both reconstructing my inner being and then finding a way to communicate the pilgrimage, so to speak. I actively learned and synthesized the information, methods, and techniques. To say I saw improvement in my life on all levels is an understatement! I had become a new version of myself. The version I'd envisioned, but even better. How is that possible? Because I was not able to aim as high as I could from my starting point. In order to expand my horizons, I needed to have a greater understanding of why I was stuck in the first place. Once I could see why my patterns of behavior were not serving me well, I could then create and manifest new thoughts and beliefs, resulting in a high-frequency, high-functioning Self. Immersing myself in this process ignited a new mindset. A new me!

Here's my story: I had an unhappy and difficult childhood. At age seventeen, I enlisted in the Air Force where I was honorably discharged at age twenty. When I arrived back home, I felt aimless and empty, especially after being in war-torn territories. I started looking for a career and had many stops and starts along the way. Nothing fit the bill, yet I truly wanted to find a place where I belonged, a place I could call home. However, by the time I was thirty-one, I had invested a lot of time in two careers that were not a good fit. In between each of these careers, I also had countless jobs.

Upon discharge from the military, I had to support my mother because her husband, my step-father, had a heart attack and could not work. He was a salesman for a clothing manufacturer, so I ended up taking over his route and learned how to present the line of dresses he represented. I stayed in the garment industry for a couple of years and, long story made short, became the MOD buyer for a twenty-three-store chain in Pennsylvania.

Eventually, I opened my own retail dress shop. Did I love it? Let's say I fell into it and was good at it. I kept the momentum of sales and retail after running my step-father's business and working as a buyer. I wasn't deeply fulfilled, but it checked enough boxes at the time.

After I had worn that career into the ground, I felt the need to explore the world. I traveled to Europe and hitchhiked around Spain. Then I went to Morocco and rented a house with two English kids I met. From there, I took a freighter out of Cadiz, Spain, to the Canary Islands where I lived in a bamboo hut I built outside of a banana plantation next to the fishing village of Arguineguín on Gran Canaria. After that experience, I returned to the United States and went back to retailing. Ready to settle down and find love, I met and married my wife.

When our first child was born, I left my job in retail where I worked as an assistant manager for one of the units of Lit Brothers—a well-known department store chain in the Philadelphia area. I switched gears and dove into the wholesale automotive industry because I didn't want to work the long hours of retail. Having a child will make you not want to work holidays and weekends!

From there, I became curious about the health food industry and got a job as a representative for a national vitamin company. Finally, I found a field that was of deep interest to me: health and wellness. Working in this industry led me to becoming a naturopathic doctor. With this new training, I learned to diagnose, treat, and—most importantly—*prevent* chronic and acute illness by supporting a person's inherent self-healing capabilities. I then started my business in 1984, and this year (in 2022) the company turns thirty-eight.

The years leading up to 1984, after leaving the military, I could not stay at a job longer than three years. The reason for this restlessness was that, regardless of the positions I was promoted to or the money I made, nothing made me happy or left me fulfilled. Dissatisfaction would always seep in, and I would move on to the next situation. (By the way, you'll learn that dissatisfaction is a pattern of behavior.)

I met a couple along my healing journey who taught me the information I am going to share with you on these pages. They helped me understand how our personal concepts, patterns of behavior, and the cycles they flow in affect our health physically, spiritually, and emotionally. Their knowledge and teachings marked a pivotal change in me and forever altered the course of my life. It improved a thousandfold. I believe it can do the same for you.

Are you ready to be more? Are you ready for health and prosperity on all levels? If so, it's time to proceed on this momentous journey.

Looking for Answers!

Have you spent a small fortune on books, workshops, seminars, lectures, and life coaches, hoping the messages you read would help you improve or radically change your life? Are you still caught up in experiencing your history "repeating itself"? Unless you intentionally reflect and assess your past, which requires an honest look at the happenings in your life, then you are at risk for recurrent, unwelcome patterns. Let me give you an example. In some relationships, there's a tendency for abuse—those who were treated poorly swore "never again" to be a recipient of harmful behavior. The reason they come to this tipping point is because something that was done or said to them was so very hurtful and detrimental to the person and/or the relationship. Being involved in chaotic and detrimental situations causes extreme emotional responses that can and do cause long-lasting frustration and pain.

In your work life, you may have had plenty of jobs. Let's say you rise up the ladder only to quit or be terminated because of one reason or another. When you quit a job, you tell yourself (and others!) there was a logical, rational, and justifiable reason for doing so. This way, the focus is taken off of you. Why would you do this? Because it's too difficult to have the self-awareness that highlight some of your faults. (This is one pattern of behavior that employs *dissatisfaction*.)

Quitting the job sets you up for additional problems, such as financial difficulties. Because of the loss of employment, you struggle to make ends meet; therefore you take another job, usually starting near the bottom, and rise up the company ladder again—only to quit before being let go for one reason or another.

Physically, there are tendencies to catch a cold, a virus, or the flu every year or so. Then there are the accidents that you'll notice occur more frequently than you'd like. The causes behind these low-vibrational situations are easily traced back to unresolved emotional issues and a lack of proper understanding of how to overcome constant physical and spiritual defeat. In other words, it's imperative to understand your patterns and your foundational beliefs.

These and other repetitive situations may have been exactly what you were trying to put an end to, yet they still remained attached to your life. So what do you do? Seek another source of guidance and understanding. The key to extinguishing your exhaustive,

Dedication

This book is dedicated to all my guides and teachers who taught me how to think in a way that allowed for deep spiritual development. They also taught me how to have eyes that see and ears that hear. My life is forever changed by what they shared with me, such as the mysteries life and how to find answers within myself.

Thanks to them, I have grown and improved myself over the years. First, I became an independent business owner and found my personal path, which then led me to peace, balance, and harmony within and without.

Table of Contents

—Always Need to be right

—Approval

—Arguing

—Being a Victim

—Comedian

—Demanding

—Denial

—Depletion

—Desperation

—Disappointment

—Dissatisfaction

—Distraction

—Embellishing

—Excess

—Fear Doubt

—Guilt

—Impatience

—Imposition

—Laziness

—Lying

—Manipulation

—Obligation

—Overcompensation

—Perfection

—Procrastination

—Rejection

—Resentment

—Sacrifice

—Savior

—Self-Destruction

—Selfishness

—Self-pity

—Success Failure

—Withdrawal

unproductive cycles is understanding! Understand why you did what you did. Also, understand why you continue to do what you do, especially if you are unfulfilled and lack drive and purpose.

I guarantee that if you apply the information contained on the following pages, there will be apparent growth, which will manifest as better health, deeper relationships, and material (financial) prosperity. Of course, your success hinges on you applying these methods and techniques on a regular basis. All it takes is seeing, listening, thinking, evaluating, and acting.

The Operating System

The operating system for any computer contains the initial setup programs that initiate other programs and software upon being started and booting up. For example, the date and time is automatically current when the screen illuminates and shows your home page. The calendar is updated, and your appointments and tasks are brought up so that you know what is ahead for the day. The daily news and weather are also current. You are now informed of the day ahead on some levels—commitments, responsibilities, and obligations. Everything is laid out so you can proceed with specific plans of action to accomplish your goals, provided nothing else occurs that will disrupt, alter, or change the predetermined schedule.

Think of the brain/mind as a computer. It has a fundamental operating system. On top of this operating system sits the software programs designed to perform specific functions, whether it is a Word document, a calculating program, or a creative presentation program. They each provide an end result the user needs or desires—all based on input. Each program responds to input and then goes into action by presenting the end result associated with that program.

Now the system is on and awake, waiting for you to give it commands.

Disciplined Approach

If you're like me, you have a disciplined approach to beginning each day. My first step when I arrive at work is to "walk the floor" and say good morning to each employee. As I walk around, I am also looking at where things stand. I do an assessment. What needs to be done? What's left over from the day before?

Once I get to my office, I automatically go through a system of tasks: I listen to voice mail. I read emails. I look at my to-do list. I prioritize the day's tasks. Then I prioritize my phone calls and emails and add them to my to-do list. By this point, I am ready to work and initiate the software programs associated with my projects and tasks. I input the information based on my walk-around.

Additional software programs are initiated based on my tasks, phone calls, and emails. With that, the day is off and running! And life goes on! After lunch, the same routine is repeated, starting with my "walk around."

The Human Operating System

The concept of a computer is based on the operations of the human brain. Here's how the mind operates: Upon falling asleep, the mind is still running programs, analyzing the events and stimuli from the day. It then creates dreams that offer insight as to which software programs were initiated, unbeknownst to you. They were seen and/or heard but did not register consciously; however, they did register subconsciously.

Examples of automatic programs that are constantly working without input are the heartbeat (circulation) and breathing (respiration). At night, the software running the repair process kicks in once you fall asleep. During these hours, your body is rebuilding some systems, creating new cells, and detoxifying the bloodstream as best it can.

Upon waking, other automatic software programs become active. Your eyes open. You get out of bed and go to the bathroom. Subroutines begin to kick in as well. You may prepare coffee or tea or pour yourself juice or milk. Then you prepare and eat breakfast. From there, it's time to clean up for the day, shower, brush your teeth, and then dress and go to work, school, or wherever the day takes you.

Obviously, some of this applies to you and some does not based on your personal reality. What's important to note are the automatic things that you did without consciously having the thought to do so.

Now that you are up and running, interacting with your significant other, parents, or children will determine which software programs will be stimulated and put into action. The human operating system can also be seen to have other pre-programmed directives—of a spiritual nature—which are based on the Universal Principles.

So that there is an understanding of the term, a Universal Principle is defined as "a fundamental truth or proposition that serves as the foundation for a system of belief or behavior, or for a chain of reasoning." A perfect example used in the dictionary is "the basic principles of Christianity." The Eightfold Path of Buddhism is another.

Jesus' teachings are also considered Universal Principles: Love God. Love your neighbor as yourself. Forgive others who have wronged you. Love your enemies. Ask God for forgiveness of your sins. Repentance of sins is essential. Don't be hypocritical (see Exodus 20:1–17; Matthew 7:5). Actions will reflect Christian virtues, such as humility, faith, charity, courage, self-government, virtue, industry, and wisdom.

The Eightfold Path is another set of Universal Principles: right understanding, right thought, right speech, right action, right livelihood, right effort, right mindfulness, and right concentration.

There are many other words that are also associated with the concept of principles. Throughout this work, I will be using the term Universal Teaching. The reason I refer to the teachings as universal is because it does not matter what your beliefs or spiritual practice may be. The teachings are based on the Immutable Laws of God and are therefore applicable to everyone.

A teaching is defined as "ideas or principles taught by an authority." The example used in the dictionary was: "the teachings of the Koran." *Teaching* can also be defined as "engagement with learners to enable their understanding and application of knowledge, concepts and processes." An example would be any craft that requires skill and attention to detail, such as cabinet makers, electricians, dental hygienists, not to mention the arts of medicine and surgery.

The Brain

The Hard Drive

The brain functions on many levels. The functions are categorized on two levels: the conscious and the subconscious. The subconscious represents the automatic functions of the brain that do not require any thought whatsoever, or any input from the mind. The brain is the housing that operates the body and, at the same, time contains the mind. *The mind influences the brain, which in turn affects the body.*

Here's a perfect example: You're driving on the highway, and the next thing you hear is a police siren. You look in your rearview mirror and the police car is flashing its lights right behind you. Upon seeing the red lights and hearing the siren, your heart begins to pound, your adrenaline is released, and you may even get a queasy feeling in your stomach. All of these reactions are based on sight and sound, including your association with authority and the police.

The mind also functions on many levels at once. Here, they are categorized on four active levels at once. The first being the aspect that is connected to the God Force that dwells within and without. Luke 17:21 says, "Neither shall they say, Lo here! or, lo there! for, behold, the Kingdom of God is within you."

The second is the unknown or the subconscious mind that contains all of the software programs of how to act and respond based on external stimuli. The third attribute is the gathering of data and input that you are not aware of. In scientific circles this is called *unconscious cognition.* This is the processing of perception, memory, learning, thought, and language without being aware of it.[1] This gathering also plays into stimulating software programs. The fourth level of consciousness is where one is expressing and actively involved in endeavors on whatever level that may be. Endeavors are the result and application of the software at work.

Deep in/on the Hard Drive

The primary directive that is buried deep within the mind, below the subconscious, is the spiritual directive to live and bring balance and harmony into everything you do. This is possible because you have dominion over everything. In Genesis 1:27–28, it says, "So God created man in his own image, in the image of God created he him, male and female

created he them. And God blessed them, and God said unto them, Be fruitful, and multiply, and replenish the earth, and subdue it, and have dominion over the fish of the sea, and over the fowl of the air, and over every living thing that moveth upon the earth."

This power of dominion is what you're supposed to exercise in the effort to bring balance and harmony into your life. You have the tools to do so: Understanding. Knowledge. Expression. Imagination. Will. Faith. Perseverance. Strength. Objectivity. Honesty. Healing. Love.

God loves active participation, not passive acceptance.

The Human Software

The way of looking at software programs in the mind is seeing them as concepts. These concepts are maintained in your subconscious mind. Like software, they influence and direct your life based on input. Concepts, like software programs, go into action when one or more are triggered through sight, sound, smell, taste, or touch. Any input into one of these senses acts as a facilitator, making a concept within aware of the need for a response. At that moment, a pre-programmed response begins its cycle. Preprogrammed responses are seen as patterns of behavior. These are created by you, in your formative years, to validate the concept as being true. Even when it is detrimental to your well-being.

Software programs for computers are created by developers who construct the software language to perform the desired results without delay or "hiccups." These programs can be altered, updated, and even overwritten by processes the developer sets in motion.

The concepts that you have acquired can also be altered, modified, and overwritten to create new results. It takes applying the knowledge gained from seeing and listening, then doing the exercises, methods, and techniques presented here.

What" we think, we become."
—Buddha

Concepts

"Visiting the iniquity of the fathers upon the children, and upon the children's children, unto the third and to the fourth generation" (Exodus 34:7). In this Universal Teaching, the iniquities that are being passed on are the concepts. These are the ideals, standards, and values that are taught to the offspring by example. The examples are given through demonstrations, acting in a particular way to each situation that arises—verbally and through attitude.

Every aspect of your life is influenced and affected by your concepts. Concepts are the guides that act as the foundation of your belief system. Your concepts are the glasses that you look through. Like rose-colored lenses, your perceptions are tinted by your belief system. You form your opinions, actions, and reactions based on that tinted perspective. Here are some very common examples of concepts that people share:

- God is a man: "So God created man in his own image, in the image of God he created him; male and female he created them" (Genesis 1:27). The part that says we are created in the image of God is our spirit, our soul. The soul is, in its natural state, genderless. The gender we are today is designed to teach us about ourselves.
- According to Aristotle's teachings, "Men create gods after their own image, not only with regard to their form but with regard to their mode of life."
- "You are born with sin." This is another great misconception. This thought is based on Eve eating the apple, and her and Adam being exiled from the garden of Eden. This is the famous "fall from grace."

Following is the Bible passage and its meaning from a different perspective. "And the woman said unto the serpent, We may eat of the fruit of the trees of the garden: But of the fruit of the tree which is in the midst of the garden, God hath said, Ye shall not eat of it, neither shall ye touch it, lest ye die" (Genesis 1:3:2–4).

It is worth recalling that the Tree of Knowledge of Good and Evil was in the middle of the garden. This symbolically tells us that deep within our center, in the deepest aspect of our subconscious mind, resides the connection with the God Force. It is when we are in touch with this aspect of our Self that we are able to master material life.

There is another aspect to this teaching. This statement tells of our descending into the material plane from a spiritual plane. If we were to have stayed on the spiritual plane, we wouldn't die. We choose to manipulate and control the energy of the material plane from within it. We chose to partake of the material, symbolically portrayed in the "eating of the apple," as a way of subduing it and bringing it under control so that the God Force could continue its journey. Because Spirit chose to enter into the material plane, it became subject to material laws. This is known as the "fall from grace."

Eve's eating the apple is the symbolic statement of our choice to enter into the material plane. It also denotes a lack of faith on our part. We chose the material over the spiritual. Some misconceptions taught by man are:

- *The white race is superior*. This is simply an egocentric perspective. The truth is, all men are created equal. It is interesting to read what Jesus taught on this matter. "That ye love one another; as I have loved you, that ye also love one another. By this shall all men know that ye are my disciples, if ye have love one to another" (John 13:34–35). There is no mention of color because there were shades of skin from deep brown to white in the country of Israel. It is highly likely that Jesus was brown-skinned.
- *Material possessions make you whole and complete*. Nothing could be further from the truth.
- *"It is easier for a camel to go through the eye of a needle, than for a rich man to enter into the Kingdom of God"* (Mark 10:25).
- *Money equals power and authority*. Here again, we see the teachings of man at work. True power and authority originate from within. It is from the God Force and God Energy that dwells within you. Here is the Universal Teaching to support this: "Neither shall they say, Lo here! or, Lo there! For, behold, the Kingdom of God is within you" (Luke 17:21).

The above concepts, and many more, are at work every day, shading and distorting your perception. This also includes the concept of who you think you are supposed to be in every situation. When a concept gets activated, you seek to validate it as being true. This is accomplished through the use of pre-programmed responses known as behavioral patterns.

In order to understand the concepts you're engaged with, it's necessary to dig into them systematically. *First, begin by listing all of the roles that you participate in.* For example, you have a role as a male or a female. Then you have a role as a friend, business owner, manger, employee, coworker, and entrepreneur. Each role carries a different set of behavioral expectations, resulting in specific patterns of behavior. And each role is built on a unique concept.

One of the hardest things for a person to do is to look within and take personal responsibility. Why? Victim mentality is easier than accountability. Playing the victim focuses on the belief (or concept) that everything that happened to them was something that couldn't be helped, couldn't be avoided, or was the result of someone's else's actions.

On top of that are other concepts that say, "You are not smart enough." "You haven't been trained. You don't know what you are doing." People are also told that they need a "professionally trained" person to help them. In some cases, a licensed counselor or a medical specialist is a good way to begin. In most cases, though, it is not necessary because you already have the best guides to uncover the answers within you. All you need to do is learn how to connect with them. Engaging in this work will show you how.

There is a method and exercise to help you become aware of the roles you act out based on the concepts you have. The place to start is your gender. How is it that you identify yourself as a male or a female? Look at the role your gender plays in your situation. These answers will be the result of first gaining insights. Insights lead to understanding. Understandings provide answers and act as the spearhead for your ability to change and improve the Self by removing your detrimental traits and habits.

Here is the exercise: On a blank sheet of paper in the left-hand column, list how effective you are as a: child, sibling, spouse, parent, aunt/uncle, cousin, or partner. For example, I might answer: *As a son, I am obedient, always doing what is expected of me. I complete all my chores and am thoughtful and caring .I provide for my parents. As a brother, I get along great with my siblings. I look out for them. I protect them. I care for them. I am their confidant. As a husband, I am thoughtful, considerate, generous, and participate in providing for the family. As a father, I seek to understand my children. I am supportive. I help with school work. I teach them different skills, like riding a bike and driving a car.*

These examples should provide you with the beginnings of a thought process. Of course, you will be adding to these activities as you dig deeper and recall all that you do in each role.

Now we go to the right-hand side of the paper where you will write down why you think the way you do. Are you emulating your father, mother, or a combination of both? Doing this exercise will show you who you emulate. Now, through observation, you will have a handle on seeing how it is you generally react, and act, in situations.

The exercise above is based on a positive relationship with your parents. There are others who do not have such a relationship. In fact, it is the exact opposite. Here are some examples of each aspect: As a son, this person has a troubled relationship with his parents. He does not do anything they ask of him. He fights with them, disobeys, or ignores their rules. As a brother, he is disagreeable with his siblings. They may have constant disagreements, fighting, or he could be indifferent. As a husband, he could be domineering, inconsiderate, selfish, always looking for what is wrong. This would also apply to his children. You can imagine the rest of the ways that he interacts with people, be it other family members as well friends and coworkers. On the job, he may not finish projects on time. He will likely make mistakes that in some way will cost the company money. And when he gets fired, in his mind there was a logical, rational, and justifiable reason why things that led up to the termination were not his fault. Even though he seeks confrontation, he still may have a friend or two who sticks by him because "birds of a feather flock together."

Take these examples and add to them as you think deeply in this realm. You can make some adjustments and apply it to all the types of roles you play in life. The role as an owner, manager, employee, or an entrepreneur are specific unto your expression of Self. What are you manifesting in the role that applies to you? Are you authoritative? Are you amiable? Are you agreeable? Are you forgiving or unforgiving? Asking yourself questions is essential. The answers pave the way for the new path you will walk, the new you that you will be presenting to your world.

Another role is that of a friend. What do you expect of others in terms of them being a friend to you? What do you expect of yourself in terms of being a friend to them? How do you manifest that? What does that look like from what you think you should be receiving and what do you think you should be giving?

These are some of the concepts to begin with, to really dig into. Whatever comes up first will be somewhat superficial. Question often and deeply. Don't accept your first answer. Why? Because the truth lies a bit deeper. Ponder these things to understand why your personal history repeats itself. Here is the Universal Teaching on this phenomenon found in Ecclesiastes 3:15: "That which hath been is now; and that which is to be hath already been; and God requireth that which is past." Every role that you play has patterns of behavior and expectations associated with it.

Patterns of Behavior

Patterns of behavior are what you create to validate the concepts you maintain in your subconscious mind. These are things you do to prove you are who you think you should be. What particular patterns do you engage in? There is a large list later in this book to help you identify those that may be a part of your life and expression.

You have a way of responding to people in a very particular fashion. There are particular patterns of behavior that you yourself institute, instigate, and apply for only one purpose: to validate the concepts you maintain in your subconscious mind. Your patternistic responses will generally be the same, whether you are male or female.

How do you know a pattern? The easiest way to look at it is as a stimulus, a transaction, and a result. In sales, there is something comparable to patterns of behavior called the sales cycle because both have a particular flow. It is all about the approach, the demonstration, and the close. When you are stimulated, it's because of something you have heard, seen, felt, tasted, or smelled. Any one of those stimulates a concept in your subconscious mind into action.

In the demonstration part in sales, it is about features and benefits. Here, you should be able to see the pattern by how you respond to the stimuli. For instance, a man may come home from work and look around the house and see something he felt should have been done but wasn't. The minute he sees that, he becomes angry: "Well, why didn't you do this? You're home all day. What's the story? You get home earlier than I do. You could have done this!"

These are the kinds of things that sometimes occur in relationships. These are also the same kinds of things that get blown out of proportion and are done in order to get a particular result. The woman may say, "Oh honey, I am so sorry. I should have done it." What needs to be understood, in this example, is that the woman *seeks rejection*. For her, his rejection is a form of love and acceptance. Acceptance which guarantees access to "the doorway home."

Here is how a person develops rejection as their mode of acceptance. There are two fundamental modes used for acceptance: approval and rejection. Rejection begins in the womb, the place of security in the soul's mind. As the soul is maturing within the womb, it is feeling its host's/mother's emotional state. This state maybe one of resentment, anger, or even obligation—just to mention a few energies that could be at work.

The reason for these energies can vary. Maybe be the mother did not want to be pregnant because of disharmony in the relationship; the house wasn't big enough for the addition of a child; she didn't feel they could afford a child; or her career was more important. All of these thoughts generated an energy that was fundamentally anger and rejection. However, because of religious reasons, she felt she could not abort the pregnancy. Therefore during the development stages, there was always a negative/ rejection energy being experienced by the developing child.

To keep the rejection going, there may have been a difficult and painful delivery. Today, this person associates rejection with "love and acceptance." As a result, in all matters of interacting, they will seek out rejection as a means of guaranteeing access to "the doorway home—"the same doorway from which they entered into this world. This doorway is also the way back to the peace and harmony of the spiritual plane.

This is further explained after the section on *expectations*. What do you do that stimulates a pattern or a reaction in someone else? Specifically, I'm referring to your partner or whomever you are spending significant time with or are living life with. Why? Because this is the person who also has compatible operating software, which is why you are together.

Expectations

Fulfilling expectations is the end goal of every pattern. Expectations are fulfilled by either attracting or repelling those energies that validate the particular pattern at work. The "energies" could be a person, an event, an accident, or physical item, such as a computer.

Since the mind is an electromagnetic generator, you will either draw to you what you need to fulfill your expectation, or you will repel something, such as opportunities, money, or even relationships. This is done in order to fulfill the expectation that you have relative to a particular concept that you maintain in your subconscious mind.

Listening to something sets in motion particular patterns. As an example, if you get reprimanded at work, you may come home and start an argument with your wife, your children, or, as the old cliché goes, "beat up the dog." When a concept in the subconscious mind is triggered by a physical attack, by something someone says to you, or by something that you see, then patterns are stimulated into action. This in order to facilitate the expectation associated with the concept that was triggered.

All of the examples, and especially a physical discomfort, are indications of energies at work. They indicate where you are in the cycle of a pattern of behavior. The Universal Teaching here is "forewarned equals forearmed." The "arming" is knowing what is going to unfold. Understanding this teaching gives you the opportunity to change an attitude. This allows you to make a healthier choice, which, in turn, can change the pre-programmed result and alter your path.

"The Doorway Home"

The question arises, "Where do these concepts come from?" The answer is simple. They come through your mom (as an example). She learned them from her mom, who learned them from her mom, and so on.

The next question is: "Why do we accept them?" Again, the answer is simple. We all want to return to the spiritual plane where it is peaceful, balanced, and harmonious—unlike here. In our deepest subconscious mind, we believe that by having our mom's acceptance, we are guaranteed a way back.

We Are Spiritual Beings in a Material Body

The way to stop passing on concepts is to identify the ones you work with, gain control over their patterns, and create a new and better you. By gaining control, you stop teaching your children by example through your language and attitudes.

An example in the Bible of concepts being passed on can be found in this Universal Teaching in Exodus 34:7: "And that will by no means clear the guilty; visiting the iniquity of the fathers upon the children, and upon the children's children, unto the third and to the fourth generation."

The Universal Teaching in Mark 3:31–35 says, "There came then his brethren and his mother, and, standing without, sent unto him, calling him. And the multitude sat about him, and they said unto him, Behold, thy mother and thy brethren without seek for thee. And he answered them, saying, Who is my mother, or my brethren? And he looked round about on them which sat about him, and said, 'Behold my mother and my brethren! For whosoever shall do the will of God, the same is my brother, and my sister, and mother."

Jesus is saying that he is no longer bound by the concepts he learned from his mother. He is a new, better person, able to manifest the power and identity of Spirit. He also taught the following Universal Teaching found in Matthew 18:3: "And said, Verily I say unto you, Except ye be converted, and become as little children, ye shall not enter into the kingdom of heaven." The meaning of this teaching is that you must become defenseless. In as much as defenses protect us from external attack, they also imprison us and prevent us from expanding our consciousness and being open to spiritual input.

The Four Selves

You have four different perspectives on life, and you react in four different ways, but always for the same purpose. You always seek to manifest your will, fulfill expectations, and validate your subconscious concepts as being true. The catch-22 is that it is your subconscious concepts may or may not be the conscious desires of what you want to accomplish.

The Four Selves are:

- The Spiritual Self
- The Emotional Self
- The Physical Self (also the Material Self)
- The Social Self

These four selves also represent the four cycles in the sense that every cycle begins in your Spiritual Self, then builds with either courage and confidence or doubt and fear. Next, you flow into the emotional cycle, then the physical/material cycle, and finally the social cycle. There are cycles within cycles. Never underestimate the power of cycles because your patterns of behavior flow in cycles.

One of my favorite passages in the Bible is Ecclesiastes 3:15. Read it, learn it, and memorize it. Why? Because it is all about patterns of behavior. To sum up this particular Universal Teaching, it says that wherever you are now, whatever it is you are doing now, you have done it before. And you will do it again in the future.

What is occurring now looks different because you are older, and the environment and situation *appear* to be different. Fundamentally, though, the energy is the same. This is why history repeats itself, as does your personal emotional history. As an example, you may say you are never going to date "that kind of person" again. You'll never put yourself in "that type of situation," and yet you find yourself there. Another part of this Universal Teaching states that the future, tomorrow, is now! Why? Because it is a pattern of behavior; it flows in a cycle.

Spiritual Self

Are you religious? Are you spiritual? Are you agnostic or atheist? Do you believe in a higher power? Do you attend church, synagogue, or a house of worship? Do you have icons that you take with you for security? Or perhaps you have a meditation or ceremonial area set up in your room with candles, religious icons, incense, and other items? If you are religious, do you question the teachings that are being said or taught? Do you find fulfillment and comfort in the messages you hear? Do your beliefs and practices give you what you want or what you need?

I hear people say, "Praise the Lord!" and "Thank Jesus!" for this and that. I wonder what they think and feel when the things they asked for were not given? Did Jesus fail them? Did God fail them by not delivering? I am sure they prayed for what they needed, wanted, or desired, so how does one determine the truth necessity of those needs?

The teachings of man would have you believe that if you pray and ask and do not get, then something is wrong with you. In some way, the person who asked may now feel they are unworthy. Not true. You are perfect. You are incredible! You may not think so. You may not believe so, but you are. You are a part of God, so how could you be less than incredible or anything less than wonderful?

We are spiritual beings in a material body.

Everything starts in the Spiritual Self. It receives directives from God. However, those directives get corrupted by the Emotional Self (ego), and that emotional energy is what alters everything.

Right now you are in the process of creating a scenario or situation to validate particular concepts. Look around and see if you can discover what energies are at work. What thoughts and emotions are stimulated? The year-end holidays, for example, stimulate feelings in lots of people. Because these feelings are going to motivate you, maybe even manipulate you, into creating desired outcomes, and the outcomes will be validations of the concepts.

Inasmuch as your mind is a creator, destruction also exists because it is the exact opposite. Balance and imbalance. Harmony and disharmony. Creation and destruction. Are you in the process of destroying something? A project, relationship, friendship, or association? If so, why? These are things to ponder.

From the same perspective, is *destruction* part of the validation process? Do you know your validation process? Do you know which particular concept is used with a particular pattern of behavior? Do you know the end results of the patterns of behavior that validate the concepts? Understanding these things is crucial to your growth.

Universal Teachings provide you with *symbols* to help you understand where you are in the cycle. By having this knowledge, you can change the outcome of any particular pattern of behavior. What is happening right now in your life? What is the reality you are creating? These questions are necessary to ask yourself because your growth hinges on your active participation.

God loves active participation, not passive acceptance.

What is your reality like now? Get four pieces of paper and label them accordingly:
- My Spiritual Self

- My Emotional Self
- My Physical Self (aka My Material Self)
- My Social Self

What is going on in each of these arenas? What concepts do you think you are presenting to the world? What concepts do you think you are defending? You are making a presentation and manifesting your concepts of who it is you think you should be. In the same regard, often you may come into a place where you have to defend who it is you think you should be.

Co-Creation

Be mindful that you are always in the process of co-creating your reality. That is why it is vital to know what is going on. There are a couple of Universal Teachings to help you understand what you are creating. One is to "know what you are looking at.[1]" When you understand what you are looking at emotionally, energetically, and symbolically, things will become clear.

In the King James Version of the Bible, it says to "know what is before your eyes and all the mysteries will be revealed.[2]" The greatest mysteries in life generally revolve around these questions: Who am I? Why am I here? Do I have a calling? If so, what is my calling? Do I have specific gifts? If so, what are my gifts? What is the real purpose of my life? What is the real purpose of life itself?

Your life is currently manifesting based on your current belief system, which is based on your level of understanding, your level of control over your emotions, and your level of self-acceptance—as well as your mastery over all things. So whatever your life is about at the moment, it is your co-creation.

There is a saying, "Be careful what you wish for because you just might get it." The reality is that what you are wishing for at a subconscious level is to maintain acceptance from Mom so you can return to the spiritual plane. Everything is motivated from the subconscious mind to keep that doorway open.

Co-Creating Reality

---

[1] Jesus said: "Know what is in thy sight and what is hidden from thee will be revealed to thee. For there is nothing hidden which will not be manifest."—*The Gospel According to Thomas* 5

[2] For there is nothing covered that will not be revealed, and hidden that will not be known.—"Matthew 10:25-27.

You are co-creating your reality. There is an expression, "Let go and let God." When you "let go," you are giving up your dominion, which was given to you in Genesis. Letting go allows your mind, your subconscious concepts, to run on automatic. That is when those concepts and their patterns are going to manifest. God is indifferent. God does not care. You have been given dominion over everything.[3] You exercise your dominion by gaining control. Passive acceptance is not the mode of the day.

You need to be an active participant in the construction of your life. If you are not, then you are living in passive acceptance, meaning you have given up direction and control and are living in the "let go and let God" mindset. Your subconscious mind and the expectations of who you think you need to be in order to maintain acceptance is in full control. Your mind is going to work to fulfill your expectations of who you think you should be because you have to validate the concepts that keep the ego alive. However, that is the last thing you want to do.

You want to come to a place of understanding so you can allow your ego to be less of a dominant force in your life. This does not mean that you need to become weaker. Not at all. You need to be stronger and develop your personal power, then walk with quiet strength in the surety of who you are as a part of the Creative Continuum called God. Remember this Universal Teaching: "The kingdom is within as well as without.[4]" By going within, you become a participant in exercising the power, rights, gifts, and abilities that you have been given as a citizen of the kingdom. Use it and more will be given.[5]

I can tell you from a life of interesting adventures and adversity, that all things can be overcome. I work from that principle . . . that whatever I am confronted with, I know I will get through it and come out on top. I know that I will survive because I have faith in Self. I know that I am a part of God. I am not asking God to do it for me because I have been given dominion over everything.

---

[3] Then God said, "Let Us make man in Our image, according to Our likeness; let them have dominion over the fish of the sea, over the birds of the air, and over the cattle, over all the earth and over every creeping thing that creeps on the earth." —Genesis 1:25-27

[4] Jesus said: "If those who lead you say to you, 'See, the Kingdom is in heaven then the birds of the heaven will precede you. If they say to you: 'It is in the sea' then the fish will precede you. But the Kingdom is within you and it is without you. If you [will] know yourselves, then you will be known and you will know that you are the sons of the Living Father. But if you do not know yourselves, then you are in poverty and you are poverty."—*The Gospel According to Thomas* 3

[5] "For to everyone who has, more will be given, and he will have abundance; but from him who does not have, even what he has will be taken away."—Matthew 25:29

The Emotional Self

Your Emotional Self (aka ego) is your subconscious and conscious mind. It is about being aware of your reality and interacting within it. Below the conscious, aware mind lives the subconscious, where unconscious thoughts germinate. These thoughts become the foundation for action and implementation to accomplish specific goals.

The Emotional Self is where concepts are created and seek acceptance from Mom. Mom was the doorway into the material plane from the spiritual plane. We do not want to be cut off from being able to return. Your Emotional Self is the Self where marketing is directed toward. Books, movies, games, everything is directed to the Emotional Self. The affirmations, enlightenment, self-realization, self-actualization, and self-gratification are all about the Emotional Self.

The Material Self

Material reality is a completely different matter. Are you part of the haves, the have-nots, or the get-bys? What is your material reality? It, too, is a reflection of your thinking. Your Material Self is tied in to your Emotional Self. Look at your life. What do you have? What do you own? What owns you? Does the bank own you? Do the credit card companies own you? Are items such as your car, business, or home paid for? Are you free and clear and answering to no one? Who are you still obligated to?

What kind of car do you drive? What color is it? Is it a sedan? Your car is also a reflection of you. How do you live? Are you like most Americans, earning $50,000 a year and living on $75,000 a year? Or are you making $75,000 a year and living on $50,000? Perhaps you earn $25,000 and are getting by on $10,000? Are you trying to prove anything? Are you trying to demonstrate that you are living up to the promise you made to your parents?

Your parents may have implied or told you that you would be rich and successful. Is that what you are striving to be? Or do you say, "I am not going to be any of those things because they are shallow. I am going to work a humble job and live simply." Do you know what is motivating you? Are you coming from approval for acceptance, or is rejection your form of acceptance? How are you living? What are you out to prove? All of this is in keeping with what it is you are here to master and learn. Sometimes it is painful, and you wish it would just all go away because you do not want to learn anything that makes you responsible for your decisions. But, no! You have work to do and deep things to understand.

The Physical Self

From the physical point of view, look at yourself. What kind of shape are you in? Tall, short, heavy, thin, sickly, robust? Are you on any medications? What is going on physically? What part of you hurts? What are you dealing with and why?

What Is Within?

Another Universal Teaching states: "What is within will manifest without." Said differently, life is built from the inside out. It could be that your bone marrow is a portal to the other side, the spiritual plane. Your marrow not only makes your blood, it also creates antibodies that protect you. Your bones, where the marrow is, symbolize your strength. Bones serve as your support system. Your blood is symbolic of spirit because it carries oxygen, and oxygen is symbolic of spirit, of God.

Immune System

Your immune system is always on guard, always ready to protect you. Some immune cells mature in the bones, others in the thymus. So from one point of view, your strength is always there, always ready to be utilized, just as the defense mechanisms are ready—both on a protective level and as a defensive posture. They do one and the same.

I chose both words because defenses, inasmuch as they protect you, also wall you in. When you are walled in, you cannot communicate outwardly. Your faith and protection reside there. You are constantly co-creating your reality. You are constantly fulfilling your expectations.

The Social Self

Your Social Self is the persona you use when you are with a handful of people. When in this mode, you draw on those concepts that tell you how to act and respond to certain stimulants. Some situations will trigger certain patterns. One such pattern may be to withdraw from the group and stand alone, resting your back against a wall. In other places, you may lose yourself in the TV, or find just one person to talk with. There are some who must be the life of the party, who draw in everyone's attention. How are you in these types of situations?

The more you know yourself, the less likely you will feel out of place or vulnerable to an outside attack. That will go a long way in not having a pattern of behavior triggered, enabling you to maintain harmony no matter what.

The Children of Darkness

You are a Child of Light. It is through your emotions and attachments that you are immersed in the material plane. Your opposites, the Children of Darkness, influence your actions through your emotional channels.

The Children of Darkness utilize emotions to stimulate destruction, disharmony, and imbalance because from a different point of view, that is their purpose. That is why the Emotional Self is so important to get under control. That is why Jesus said to "offer the other cheek.[6]" If a guy hits you and you hit him back, you are going to continue to fight. If you go there, it is going to get out of control. Someone is going to pull a knife or a gun, resulting in injury or death. Turn the other cheek.

Another Universal Teaching says, "Resist not evil.[7]" The more you resist something, the more life and energy you give it. However, if you do not resist, the energy is like water and will flow over you and past you. It has nowhere to take root and take hold.

---

[6] "To him who strikes you on the *one* **cheek**, offer the other also."—Luke 6:29

[7] "I tell you not to **resist** an **evil** person."—Matthew 5:39

Signs

Seeing

Jesus said: "Know what is in thy sight and what is hidden from thee will be revealed to thee. For there is nothing hidden which will not be made manifest." This is presented in *The Gospel According to Thomas* 5. In the New Testament it is stated as: "Fear them not therefore: for there is nothing covered, that shall not be revealed; and hid, that shall not be known" (Matthew 10:26; Luke 12:2).

It is said, "You see what you want to see." There is truth in this saying because oftentimes, what you see fits perfectly well with your concepts and expectations. It also indicates that you are looking through jaded eyes. The expectation a person seeks validates a particular concept or group of concepts.

Seeing is based on the scientific principle that everything is made of atoms, which are the basic unit of material matter. Atoms contain either a positive or a negative electrical charge. These electrical charges create a magnetic force. That magnetic force is a form of energy. That magnetic energy of a particular atom will draw to it other atoms. Once they are together, they bond to each other. That aggregation is the beginning of building molecules, which can also bond together and become a material manifestation, a "thing."

Those "things," once assembled into a physical item, can become anything, up to and including a human being. Whatever the form of creation (the object), it was first a thought before it was made into form. Of course, some things are made as a byproduct of another transaction with the intent (or not) of creating a new something. Sometimes a child is the result of such transactions.

Seeing is the ability to understand the thought behind the creation of the object. This is essential in the quest for true self-knowledge as well as growth. In learning to see, your mind will draw your attention to an object in order to help you understand what you are going through at the moment. This is based on a behavioral point of view of "history repeating itself." Here is a Universal Teaching on patterns of behavior that are *not* changed found in Ecclesiastes 3:15: "That which hath been is now; and that which is to be hath already been; and God requireth that which is past." This relates to karma.

Seeing what you are looking at, and understanding what it means to you, will give you a look at which concept is at work. Let me share some examples to give you insight as to how this process works.

It's ten o'clock at night, and your teenage child is out and about. The phone rings and immediately the first thing that goes through your mind is, *Oh my god! What happened?* This thought occurs because who calls at ten o'clock at night? This only happens when there's a problem! So again, there's an emotional and physiological response to hearing the sound of the phone ringing.

Having an accident is another form of communication. Assuming it's a car accident, you ruminate on how you could have left three minutes earlier or three minutes later, which would've avoided the collision. Then the accident would not have happened. Another kind of an accident is when you cut your finger or close the car door on your hand. These actions and consequences are your mind's way of telling you something is amiss. You need to pay attention!

Everything that happens to you needs to be examined from a "signs" point of view. If you had a car wreck, or even a flat tire, it needs to be examined. Questions need to be asked. Which tire went flat? Was it the right side? Left side? Front or rear?

Here is what this particular example is telling you. If it was your front tire, it represents being stopped or thwarted from going forward with your expression. A car is a vehicle of expression because it takes you from place to place, just as your expressions move you forward—be it writing, painting, music, whatever you employ as an expressive way of being.

If it's a back tire, it represents stopping you from having the momentum to go forward. This may be because you do not have the resources to continue your forward movement. Then you need to add into the equation whether it was the right side or left side. The right side deals with faith in Self. The left side deals with monetary considerations.

These are the signs that your mind uses to tell you what's going on and serves to guide you accordingly when you understand and apply the insights. When these signs are ignored, things will continue to unfold. Your mind will then give you other signs and indications that things are amiss. Again, if not read, not worked with (dreams are one example), then something will happen to you of a physical nature. You may get a paper cut at work. You may get an infection. You may have inflammation manifest somewhere in your body. If it's not dealt with and understood, that inflammation, which is known to corrupt cells, has the potential to alter your DNA. Now you begin to set other potential problems into action. They would be appropriate for what your mind was trying to tell you. The end result could be a condition or disease.

Visual Signs

Seeing the signs are akin to looking at road signs on the highway, or a sign in your neighborhood. When you see a stop sign, you know that at the end of the street, you need to stop. This action can protect from being hit by vehicles coming from either side of you. This example is just one of many traffic signs that guide you on an accident-free journey —usually. Your mind also uses signs to help guide you. In this case, the signs tell you which pattern of behavior is going to start (and when), or where you are in the cyclic flow of it. Because of patterns and their cyclic flow, we have the Universal Teaching that says, "History repeats itself."

Another facet of your mind when seeing is it "looks back" to see how you handled a particular situation in the past. In the present moment, the situation may look entirely different; however, from the energetic and emotional point of view, it is the same as before. The same pattern is at work once again, repeating your history. Here is another Universal Teaching in regard to this theme: "Look back in order see ahead." If you have an upcoming project or something you want to work on, look to your past when you did something similar. Each of you have particular strengths, and each of you have past successes to draw on. Even when you are confronted with something that you are unfamiliar with, something that is going to trigger doubt or fear, you have successes to draw upon.

How you approach situations that appear to be new or different from past experiences is to do meditations or "program" your mind in this way: "Mind, draw on the past success that relates to this project." When you run this type of program, your mind is going to scan back to your past successes, and it will do different things for you simultaneously. One, you are now working from a position of courage and confidence versus doubt and insecurity. Your mind can draw on a past success: "I have done this before. Maybe not exactly like this, but close enough that I can handle it. I know I can do this because I have done it before." In order to draw upon a success, your mind will begin to position your perception, your understandings, and your insights, then congeal circumstances to create a reality that will allow the fulfillment and the success to manifest. Every thought has energy and reality; you are co-creating your reality as you are moving through the material plane.

If you are sending out the energy of doubt and fear, then you are attracting certain elements that are going to aggregate into a situation. But if you are drawing on courage and confidence, you are going to attract different elements. You are going to attract a different configuration in your life and have a different result.

The way to understand and work with signs is to create your own personal dictionary. For instance, in the example above about the police car and authority, you might have a page for "authority" if that is something you have issues with. As you are moving through life, there are other signs of authority that you have that, once you become aware, will become items in your dictionary. So as time goes on, you will know those signs that signal the pattern of attracting authority to you is unfolding. The reason for this is because you may draw authority to you in order to shut you down and stop your forward movement.

If you have ever been in an accident when someone else was driving, then being a passenger can make you very uncomfortable. So when a vehicle speeds up, it triggers fear that the driver may lose control or may not be able to react fast enough if a situation arises. In this example, there are multiple signs that your mind may use to tell you that a loss of control may be in the making. The signs here are the speeding, the type of vehicle, the driver, the road conditions. You only need to read one sign to know that the possibility is unfolding.

Signs are also like apps and icons, in addition to road signs. The icons that show up in your patterns are the icons that you need to learn and include in your dictionary. They become your primary source of guidance when seeing. I have learned to call them symbols.

Aromatic Signs

Smelling is yet another way that your mind talks to you. You may walk into a store and smell something your mother or grandmother made for you. It brings back specific memories. Some good, some bad. As an example, one smell might bring warm and fuzzy feelings to the surface. It may be the smell of a fabulous dinner when things were great. Everyone there had a good time. The conversation was enlightening, and your world was perfect.

On the other hand, the aroma could be associated with imposition. Maybe it was a meal that you didn't like—even though your mom, dad, or grandparents loved it. Yet to you, it did not taste good. However, you were forced to eat it or be punished. Today, that aroma implies punishment. Your mind uses these techniques to talk to you and help you get on (and keep on) the right path.

Listening Signs

Sounds trigger a feeling deep within. Sometimes that feeling is recognized as being a stimulant. Your response will be determined based on what you hear or what is said. The words could trigger feelings of inadequacy, fear, and/or anger.

Sometimes a song will come on the radio, be featured in a movie, or sound throughout a restaurant. It does not matter where or when you hear it. What matters is how you respond to the song. You may not respond right there in that moment. It may bring back a favorite memory instantly. Unbeknown to you, though, it is also triggering a concept in your subconscious mind.

The concepts that are being stimulated and the patterns they set in motion is what is important. When you have a strong reaction to a song, or something someone says to you, you do need to question it. When was this song popular? What were you going through? Who were your friends at the time? These are the types of questions that should be asked to understand which emotions have been triggered and which particular pattern of behavior is being set in motion.

Moving Forward

Listening

Lao Tzu was quoted as saying, "Silence is a source of great strength." Listening is another one of those skills necessary for growth. The reason is because anything that is said to you and anything that you hear is the manifestation of a thought. This indicates that there is an energy and intent behind what you just heard. Whereas an object, or a solid manifestation such as a sound, is a vibratory presentation. Either way, you need to understand what's being said. What is the thought behind the comment? When someone makes a joke at your expense, it's not a joke; it's an attack. When you make a joke about yourself, that is a form of denigration. Where this stems from needs to be understood. Remember: we tend to hear what we want to hear.

Listening sets in motion a specific concept and its associated patterns of behavior within the subconscious mind. The pattern of behavior begins to manifest. For example: You get hollered at work by your boss. You then come home and holler at the kids. The kids carry on the cycle by beating the dog.

Thinking

Having eyes that see and ears that hear provides you with an enormous amount of guidance in the form of information. That information is centered upon helping you understand where you are in a particular pattern of behavior. The Universal Teaching found in Ecclesiastes 3:15 says, "That which hath been is now; and that which is to be hath already been; and God requireth that which is past." This helps to explain how all patterns of behavior flow in cycles. If there is not an awareness, an understanding, and an effort to alter or control the pattern of behavior, then it repeats itself. This is echoing your personal history. Buddha's wise words caution our thinking patterns: "What we think we become."

As you can see in Ecclesiastes 3:15, patterns of behavior do not change unless you understand and take control of them. Left on their own, they will repeat. This is why the saying, "Let go and let God" is not a healthy thing to do. Lao Tzu taught, "Mastering others is strength; mastering yourself is true power." So now that you have gathered some of the information and evaluated the emotional associations you have with the objects, the person, the experience, and/or the thoughts, sounds, or things that were said to you by others, it's time to examine which ones triggered an emotional response. That emotional response, evolving from the particular concept, stimulated patterns of behavior into action.

Pondering those responses will give you insight as to how you instinctively react. The goal here is to alter your reactions. Making them more in harmony will provide you with a peaceful experience, whatever the transaction may be. What is meant by that statement is you can either get stressed out by something that stimulates doubt or fear or aggression, or you can understand it and control your emotional responses so that there is no outburst and no loss of control.

I am sure you have seen situations or been involved in one where the other party became emotional and to some degree may have said things or done things that can never be taken back. Something said or done was very hurtful to either you or the other person. Emotions that are out of control lead to chaos. It is each individual's responsibility to go back to the primary directive, which is to seek balance and harmony in any situation. Jesus said: "Whoever knows the All but fails [to know] himself lacks everything." This Universal Teaching is presented in *The Gospel According to Thomas* 67. Knowing others is intelligence; knowing yourself is true wisdom.

Evaluating

Now that you have this information and you've been pondering it, hopefully on paper so that you have references and you can organize it accordingly, it's time to make an evaluation that will lead you to a plan of action.

When you can identify a particular concept at work and its corresponding patterns of behavior, then, like any programmer, you need to rewrite the software. You need to create a new and more positive, beneficial, and harmonious program leading to a better outcome. As you are rewriting the software, instead of responding in the way that you normally would to a particular stimulus, try to understand what's going on. Understanding and pausing gives you the opportunity to apply a different response that will create a different outcome—thus creating a new "software" program. That fundamental approach begins to change how you respond to specific stimuli. Doing this helps you grow and gain control over your emotional responses, allowing you to move forward on every level from a position of personal power with quiet strength.

Acting

Acting is being. The goal is to be the person you want to be. Keep in mind this is *not* an overnight accomplishment. Do not think that because you have read this material you have suddenly mastered it. That attitude will lead to the same ole same ole. In fact, that thinking may be exactly why your previous attempts at true change and improvement may not have brought you any closer to your goals. Of course, the program may have been an intellectual effort and not a true substantive knowledge base with applicable methods and techniques. Only you know the truth of these statements.

Reprogramming Patterns

In order to reprogram your automated responses to stimuli, you first need to identify *all* the patterns of behavior you currently are using. There are over thirty patterns of behavior in use by people. Of course, not all will apply to you. Throughout this chapter I present a list of patterns, along with questions as to how you may employ them if a pattern is applicable to you. Ponder and explore the ones that speak to you so that you come to an understanding of what types of life situations and emotional states you are manifesting, because all of it is coming from you.

Programming is reinserting a new directive into your human software to override your previous program and instill different expectations in the future. Remember, the mind is goal-driven. It seeks to fulfill expectations. The way to innate programming is from the relaxed state of mind. Once deeply relaxed, you simply repeat the phrase you want to accomplish. (I have an audio available to help you with relaxation. Send an email to me at DrM@michaelshealth.com. In the subject line, type: "Relaxation.") You can create your program based upon what you need to achieve. Here are few to start with:

I am (one of the names of God), becoming aware of guidance indicators and guidance signs. I am completing my tasks in a timely manner. I am reaping the benefits of success. I am getting better at my craft.

Awareness Control
Repeat this verse from Matthew 7:7 to remind you of the power in asking: "Ask, and it shall be given you; seek, and ye shall find; knock, and it shall be opened unto you. For every one that asketh receiveth; and he that seeketh findeth; and to him that knocketh it shall be opened."

Making a List
Reprogramming is a very critical aspect of the efforts to becoming a "better, new you." The list will evolve from the examination of the following patterns of behavior that we will explore together. As we go through them, I will give you things to look for, to "see." Things to listen for and things to think about. In each section there are signs that will spark your awareness as you begin the understanding of Self. Others will be signs telling

you when a particular pattern is beginning to emerge. Knowing these things before the pattern becomes the automatic, built-in response will give you the opportunity to change the habitual outcome and truly solidify the foundation of becoming the you that you want to be.

Patterns of Behavior

The patterns of behavior listed in this section are presented in no particular order. As stated earlier, many will not be applicable to you; however, many others will. Be honest with yourself if you truly want to evolve to the next level of being. Each pattern of behavior will detail the seeing, listening, and thinking aspect to reflect on. Then you will be provided affirmations to help you reprogram a new pattern. From there, you will be asked to reflect on specific questions regarding how a specific pattern plays out in the various Selves: emotional, physical, material, social, and spiritual.

ALWAYS BEING LATE

This is another one of those patterns grown out of the need for rejection. In this scenario, the title speaks for itself. Of course, there is always a very good reason. However, the bottom line is this person actively seeks rejection. Another pattern that comes into play is that of being a victim. "I would have been here on time except on my way I was . . ." A significant consequence of this pattern is missing out on opportunities for growth and advancement. This can also tie into the patterns of denial, deprivation, and depletion. Being late more times than is acceptable could result in being terminated from employment, setting in motion the above-mentioned patterns.

Seeing

In this pattern it's more like not seeing. Not looking at the clock to check timing. It's leaving things that need to be handled in the here and now to the last minute. It's not being prepared. "Oh, I had to stop for gas, so that's why I am late." As you can see, there are contributing patterns here as well: procrastination, distraction, and a lack of preparation. The mind of this person is giving them signs that they need to get going; however, there is always one more thing to do before they leave. It's the one thing that is the stimulus to set the need for rejection in motion.

Listening

This is another one of those instances where the mind talks to the person. "Dinner is scheduled to be served at seven p.m. You have to be there in thirty minutes. Clean up and go." The other voice says, You got time. It only takes five minutes to get there, even when you know it's a fifteen-minute drive when the traffic is lite. Since the goal, rejection, is at work, along with the other patterns mentioned, someone may say something to you that sounds like a good idea and has to be done now! This triggers distraction, which is another "tool" in the arsenal of seeking rejection, hindering growth and advancement.

Thinking

When you become aware of the thoughts that are setting the stage for being late, that is your sign that the pattern is being activated. When you find yourself being distracted is another sign. In order to overcome this pattern, it takes an exerted effort to be mindful. It is necessary to take into consideration the thoughts and feelings of others. The goal here is to understand the need for rejection because it plays a major part in your expression.

Program

I am on time for appointments. I am mindful of others. I am considerate.
I am better at time management. I am not the center of the Universe.

How does this pattern play out in the various Selves?
Emotional Self
Do you set the stage for rejection?
How do you make others be late?
Physical Self
Have dinners been ruined because of you being late?
Material Self
Have you lost opportunities because of being late?
Have you lost money?
Social Self
What benefits do you derive from being late?
Do you become the center of attention when you are late, even if it's negative attention?

ALWAYS NEED TO BE RIGHT

All of us have had "discussions" with this type of person. Sometimes we think of them as the "know it all," or they admit, "I'm just being the devil's advocate." No matter how they present it, or how you think about it, they always walk away from the discussion as being right. On occasion, sometimes they may come back and say that you were right. They may even apologize.

Seeing

Always needing to be right is another one of those hard-to-see patterns at work within oneself. It is more a listening and knowing than seeing. However, there may be signs, such as "bumping" into an old acquaintance at a store or receiving a phone call or an email from them. When questioning when and what was going on in your life at the time, it could be an indication that your need to be right is manifesting, or beginning to. In this situation, you need to look at what is currently going on, where you are in it, and with whom. Oftentimes, there are certain people who stimulate you into the pattern of being right. Seeing that it's about to arise, or that you are already into it, gives you the opportunity to exit, to change a position, and drop the need to be right.

Listening

This is much easier, assuming you are listening to the things you say. It is also easier to see and hear when another person is right. Listening to what you say to others is essential if you are determined not to attack another person. Here is a Universal Teaching on this matter: "What you say is what defiles you." This is an adaptation of: "There is nothing from without a man, that entering into him can defile him; but the things which come out of him, [spoken word] those are they that defile the man" (Mark 7:15). Oftentimes, the person with this pattern will defend their position with power by being loud and overbearing. This is an indication that they are coming more from doubt than a strong knowledge-based foundation.

Thinking

This is strictly an internal questioning that must take place. In all thinking processes, it is necessary to ask questions. However, these should be directed inward to understand why you might have the need to be right all the time, regardless of the subject matter. This person will sometimes come to conclusions based on partial information combined with preconceived ideas as to how it should be, or how it should unfold. Therefore their preconceived idea is believed to be the right one.

Program

I am listening more to what others are saying. I am thinking more and speaking less.

I am no longer dealing with the need to be right all the time.

How does this pattern play out in the various Selves?
Emotional Self
Do you need to win every argument?
Is it your way or the highway?
Physical Self
Do you have set beliefs as to how things should be done?
Material Self
Do you believe that money, power, and authority over others makes you right?
Social Self
Do you pick and choose who, what, where, and when?
Spiritual Self
Do you need others to believe as you do?

APPROVAL

Approval and rejection are the two foundational modes of expression. In this pattern, the daughter is just like Mom. The boy is just like Dad. Both of these modalities are designed for the child to have his or her mother's acceptance. This is what we discussed in "the doorway home." Every concept in the subconscious mind is based on the need for acceptance from their mother. This need is so great that on some levels it stymies true growth. It prevents self-exploration and the manifestation of the desire to be more. Some children desire to step outside the family traditions, culture, and expectations but are afraid they will be rejected. This fear of rejection and need for approval cuts them off from "the doorway home."

Seeing

With the approval pattern, it is very easy to see, hear, and think about how to be compliant, how to gain approval, and how to maintain acceptance in every situation that arises. It is also easy to see this in others. The hardest thing about this pattern is the need for acceptance and the fear of rejection.

You may have family members who strive for rejection. That is their ticket home! If you have siblings, I will guarantee that when you all get together and discuss Mom and Dad, it will be as if some of you grew up in a different house with a different set of parents. On some levels, this is true. The reason for this surrounds each birth, the soul within each fetus, and the concepts the soul needs to learn and master in this life cycle. Every incarnation is a step toward mastery when one breaks from the need for approval or rejection as their form of acceptance.

Listening

Learning to listen to yourself is an important tool in gaining mastery over your emotions. In seeking approval, there are certain words that you use to acquire it. By learning what they are, you can begin to control your speech so that you approach conversations from a neutral place—place of quiet strength. This also provides you with personal power because you are not seeking approval from anyone. Another aspect to listening is hearing how others are seeking your approval. This also influences how you respond to them. And it may even stimulate your seeking for approval.

Thinking

On one level, you now know you seek approval for acceptance. So the issue becomes: How does this need this affect my thinking? Because how you think will also affect your actions and reactions. You may become, or already are, compliant to those who would dominate you. Going with the flow through compliance is a pattern of behavior. It may be that in some situations you don't want to participate, but the need for approval is so embedded that you feel obligated, which is another pattern of behavior. Now it is essential that you understand how being compliant and feeling obligated affects your life in your quest for approval.

Program

I am no longer seeking acceptance. I am becoming the person I want to be. I am getting stronger. I am becoming my true Self.

How does this pattern play out in the various Selves?
Emotional Self

Are you always willing to be or do what others want?

Do you willingly sacrifice your well-being to please others?

Do you have a need for approval?

Physical Self

Is your motto "work harder"?

Do you intentionally choose difficult jobs or volunteer for difficult tasks?

Material Self

Do you feel you must have the newest, shiniest "whatever"?

Social Self

Do you feel you must be politically correct?

Do you feel you must be the center of attention?

Spiritual Self

Do you feel an obligation to attend religious services?

ARGUING

This person is also called the "pot stirrer." There are some folks who love a good argument. Arguing can be a great tool for accomplishing many different goals. One of the first that comes to mind, though, is rejection. In this scenario, it really does not matter the context of the conversation. The person with this need will find a point of contention, or extrapolate one based on some obscure perspective.

Another aspect of arguing is tied into the "always being right" pattern of behavior. No matter what is being said or done, they are right. That does not necessarily mean that you are wrong. It's just that in their mind, they are right too. Dominance, manipulation, and obligation are other patterns that can also be drawn upon in this patternistic approach to some situations.

Seeing

It is so much easier to see the trait of arguing in someone else than it is to see it in ourselves. In fact, it is easier to see everything that is "not right" with others than it is to look at ourselves. If you are prone to getting into arguments, then it is incumbent upon you to learn the visual signs that will draw you in. Getting into arguments means that you are amenable to that occurring in your life. So to get a handle on your temper and remove this energy from your file, you need to see it coming from within as well as from without. An example might be that someone you are riding with drives in a way that you feel is dangerous or inconsiderate, such as speeding. Using the same example, you may be the driver and the passenger takes tissues with the way you drive. Arguments also evolve out of the defenses. If a person feels that they are being attacked for any reason, they may use arguing to prove they are right and you are wrong.

Listening

You can always tell when there is an argument. The volume is much higher than in a normal speaking voice. It is as if yelling will make the point clearer. It is also a sign that anger is brewing. This is why sometimes negative situations are the result of arguing. One such result can lead to death of one of the people arguing. It is vital to control your emotions, not only in this pattern but in all because the potential for ruination is great. Here are a few Universal Teachings that exemplify this understanding.

"You will not be punished for your anger,
you will be punished by your anger."
—Buddha

"Holding on to anger is like drinking poison
and expecting the other person to die."
—Confucius

"And unto him that smiteth thee on the one cheek
offer also the other."
—Luke 6:29.

"But I say unto you, That ye resist not evil;
but whosoever shall smite thee on thy right cheek,
turn to him the other also."
—Matthew 5:39.

Thinking

If arguing is part of your personality, you would benefit from asking yourself, "What do I get out of arguing?" "What purpose does it serve?" and "Why do I feel the need to present or defend my perspective?" Asking yourself questions is one of the best things you can do in becoming the person you want to be. The questions you ask relate to who you are now, so in asking you begin to gain insight as to why an argumentative nature is a part of you. Like many other patterns of behavior, this is a learned trait. In order to let go of who you think you should be and how you should act, react, and live, you need to first understand the whys behind your behavior. Once this is accomplished, then you can begin to exercise control by letting go of that which works against your spirit. From this point, becoming who you truly want to be will be easier to manifest.

Program

I am avoiding arguments. I am aware of when someone is starting an argument. I am controlling my emotional responses. I am no longer open to being baited into arguments.

How does this pattern play out in the various Selves?

Emotional Self

What does being argumentative do for you?

How does being argumentative make you feel?

What is the goal with arguing, outside of rejection?

Remember: all patterns are based on specific concepts.

Physical Self

This application is where bullying occurs and where a person uses force.

Do you use intimidation?

Material Self

Are you always looking for a better deal?

Are you always arguing, trying to get what you want on the material/physical level?

Social Self

Do you argue to gain presence?

To gain attention?

To be an authority?

Spiritual Self

Do you argue with yourself about the existence of God?

Do you feel that religion has failed you?

Do disagree on what is being taught or presented?

BEING A VICTIM

In this pattern, the person is always being taken advantage of. Often, something hurtful will occur, such as an attack, accident, or a loss (of money, a business, or a relationship). However, it is never their fault; others are doing this to them. They are the "victim."

Seeing

This pattern, like every other, flows in a cycle. So the object here is to see what the signs are pointing to: being taken advantage of; losing something valuable, such as a friend, a relationship, a job, a business. Your mind is always communicating with you, providing signs, hints, and sometimes a very direct indicator that you are going to be taken advantage of.

A great example is seeing someone at a store that you have not seen in year. Another sign may be getting a phone call from a very old acquaintance, or an email from someone you haven't seen or heard from in years. The last time you saw and interacted with this person it cost you something: Money. A friendship. A relationship. When you have an experience of this kind, don't dismiss it. Your mind drew that person to you to tell you what is in motion. Knowing that gives you the opportunity to scan your reality and see what the odds are of finding yourself as a victim, once again.

Listening

There will be things said to you that will set you up for becoming a victim. Someone may ask a favor that you are willing to do because it sounds easy and doable, yet once you embark on that course of action, things are not what was presented, and you become the "fall guy." You are responsible for the negative outcome. It's your fault. Thus, you are the victim of a thoughtful effort on your part, yet it ended badly with you being on the short end of the stick.

Thinking

Here, you must go within and ponder the things you do that create situations where you end up as the victim. An example might be where you volunteer to help someone out. They take you up on your offer, but somehow it ends up costing you money. Sometimes there are other ramifications, such as losing a job or a relationship. Another example is not taking care of something that is not working right. You let it go for one reason or another, and it ends up costing you much more than it would have if you'd dealt with it at the time it malfunctioned.

Victimhood and self-pity can go hand in hand. They both share the same concepts. One being that you are not strong enough to deal with life from a position of strength. Another aspect of thinking is seeking to discover the concept that uses this pattern as a means of maintaining access to "the doorway home."

Program

I am becoming more aware of what is going on around me. I am more aware of what someone is trying to get from me. I am no longer open to being a victim.

How does this pattern play out in the various Selves?

Emotional Self

In what situations do you feel like a victim?

Do you feel you are always being taken advantage of?

In what way do you make others into victims?

Physical Self

Do you draw physical troubles to yourself?

Were you born with or did you develop a physical condition?

Is it a genetic or hereditary disease?

Material Self

In what ways are you a victim?

How do you create situations to make yourself a victim?

Remember: the patterns of depletion come into play here.

Social Self

Are you always being taken advantage of? How do you set that up?

Do you volunteer to help and aren't appreciated?

Do you lend money to a friend or family member without getting repaid?

Spiritual Self

Do you feel that God is punishing you? If so, what for?

How is the idea of divine punishment manifesting in your life?

Do you have to sacrifice your life to care for another?

COMEDIAN

This pattern uses humor as a way of expressing oneself. It is a way of escaping punishment. Of course, this depends entirely on the household they were raised in. We learn early in our life how to push our parents' buttons to get the response we want, even if it's anger. Sometimes we also stimulate one of our siblings or friends into anger. Then when the button is pushed and sets in motion an angry reaction, the "pusher" resorts to humor to avoid the consequences of their action.

It is also a way of being the center of attention, which satisfies the need to be seen. On some levels this is a form of validation. Yes, I exist. Yes, I am recognized. Yes, they love me! The down side to this pattern is when humor is used as an attack against others, and especially self. This is a telltale sign that the person is not happy with who they are. They are denigrating themselves.

Seeing

This is a very easy pattern to see in action. The hard part is stopping oneself from indulging in this pattern. There is an element of being attuned to opportunities, although they are not used to one's benefit. Here, the awareness is used to create a "funny" thing to say or do. Because of the person's need to be funny, they may miss the opportunity for growth and advancement.

Listening

The comedian has hyper-listening that is directed, like radar, to listen for a chance to interject humor into a conversation, or another person's presentation. They may even be alone and either have a big smile on their face or burst out laughing. They are reliving and rethinking something that happened in the past.

Thinking

This is a must if a person is seeking to grow. The thinking here is to the real why. Why do I need to be a comedian? Why do I use humor? What is the concept behind this? When did this begin in my life? As you can see, in the thinking process, the greatest question is why! One must continually ask that of themselves if they truly want to evolve into the next level of consciousness and awareness. This is not to say that they should become humorless and completely detached. One needs humor in their life because "laughter is the best medicine."

Program

I am controlling my need to be the center of attention. I am controlling my attacking of others with humor. I am no longer making fun of myself.

How does this pattern play out in the various Selves?
Emotional Self
Why do you feel that you must entertain others?
Why do you make fun of yourself?
In what ways do you attack others as a "joke"?
Physical Self
In what ways do you entertain?
Material Self
What types of jokes and pranks do you perform?

Have you cost others money because of your pranks?

Social Self

Are you the life of the party? Why?

Spiritual Self

Can you find humor in things?

DEMANDING

"It's my way or the highway" is the statement associated with this pattern. It's all about attitude. This pattern centers around self-importance. I am in charge. I am the one of authority. My needs are greater than yours and need to be satisfied first. It is part of the "it's all about me" mindset. This is a pattern where the person has not done anything of consequence to gain others' respect or admiration. Therefore, they are not really inclined to do this person's bidding. So, the individual uses power and authority to demand respect and allegiance. This is the pattern of a petty tyrant. It is also used in subtle manners in every arena of a person's life and is often overlooked and dismissed as a personality trait.

Seeing

This is an easy pattern to see in operation. One important indicator is when people are in fear of the consequences of not fulfilling the person's wants, needs, or desires. It is as if the person has a sword over their head. Seeing this at work within the Self is difficult. Most people do not want to think of themself as being inconsiderate of others. Everything is good as long as the person is being served, admired, and respected, even when it is not true.

Listening

It is easier to hear this pattern at work. One part of the mind, the spiritual aspect, will tell the person, "You are stepping over the line." "You are asking too much with your entitled attitude." The ego will say, "You are wonderful. People should do what you want." "You are entitled." It is the entitlement that holds the underlying feelings of self-importance that drives this behavior.

Thinking

In the effort to grow out of this insecure and undeserving behavior, one must ask: "Why do I demand that people do things for me? Who did I learn this from?"

Program

I am asking people for help when I need it. I am no longer demanding attention. I am no longer demanding admiration. I am no longer demanding respect. I am earning respect.

How does this pattern play out in the various Selves?

Emotional Self

In what ways do you feel entitled? Why?

What do you expect from others?

Physical Self

Are you demanding of others? In what ways?

What do you expect from others?

Material Self

Do you want/need/expect/demand more in compensation for your efforts?

What do you expect from others?

Social Self

In group and social situations, what is it you demand or seek from Self and others?

Spiritual Self

What do you expect from God/Jesus/Buddha?

What do you demand of others in regards to religion?

DENIAL

This pattern often accompanies depletion. The difference is that in depletion, you have resources starting out, then through actions taken, you end up with limited resources or, in the worst-case scenario, nothing at all. In denial, you don't pursue anything that would provide you with a strong foundation to build upon. So in the end, you have nothing to lose. Denial works on multiple levels. It affects your spiritual, emotional, physical, material, social, and intellectual self. The concepts behind this particular pattern are the feelings/thoughts of not being worthy of having the good things in life. Your past actions may not allow you to feel entitled or deserving of having anything that would bring you happiness and joy. One such result might also be poor health.

Seeing

One example might be not following through on something that you knew would benefit you. Because you did not move on it, you lost an opportunity to grow and move forward. When something is offered and you don't accept it, it will be for one of many justifiable, rational, or logical reasons. One such reason might be that it is not in keeping with your style, color, price range, etc. You can see the rationale at work here. The end result is that you deny yourself something, be it a pleasure, benefit, gift, or reward.

Listening
Listening in this pattern is the same as discussed in many others. One voice will be telling you to "take it" because it will be good for you. It could help you grow. It could assist you in being healthier, more financially secure." The other voice says, "No, you don't need it," even if at some level you want or desire it.

Thinking
Like every pattern, thoughts must be directed to becoming aware of when this pattern becomes active. In the seeing and listening aspects, your mind will give you clues, emotional feelings/thoughts. At that moment, you need to stop and evaluate what is going on. "Why do I feel this way? Why am I rejecting this opportunity?" It may also be that because of the patten, you don't see an opportunity. Concepts and their pattens shade your perception and influence your thinking. Another aspect of thinking is seeking to discover the concept that uses this pattern as a means of maintaining access to "the doorway home."

Program
I am entitled to have what I need, want, and desire. I am worthy of having joy, peace, and great health. I am deserving of having the best of everything. I am open to new opportunities to grow.

How does this pattern play out in the various Selves?
Emotional Self
In what ways do you deny yourself emotional comfort?
In what ways do you deny emotional comfort to others?
What could be the ramifications of that action?
Physical Self
In what ways do you know you deny yourself physical pleasure?
Physical exercise?

Physical health?

Material Self

In what ways do you deny yourself material rewards for jobs well done?

Do you break or lose things that give you pleasure?

Do you not replace things?

How do you deny others?

What are the consequences of denying others material things?

Social Self

What do you do that ends up denying you a social life?

Have you created habits that create social rejection?

Do you deny your partner or children from having a social life?

Spiritual Self

In what ways do you think you have denied your spiritual growth?

In what ways do you think you have denied your partner or your children's spiritual growth?

In what ways do you deny yourself spiritual growth with the belief that you are being religious?

DEPLETION

This particular pattern is one that leads to the loss of resources, whether it be money, material possessions, or health. There are other patterns that may have similar results when activated, but they don't necessarily cost you your security. This pattern borders on the concepts of being unworthy, incapable, and possibly needing rejection. In this aspect, it is a matter of not being successful. If one were to be successful, it would deny them the ability to return to the spiritual dimension. Being denied access to "the doorway home" is the goal when people seek rejection. The success/failure pattern was the first pattern we discussed. As you can see, it has far-reaching tentacles that affect many aspects of a person's life and well-being.

Seeing

Here are a few examples of actions that people take that deplete their money. Gambling is a great example. It is done in hopes of winning large sums of money. The reality, in most instances, is they lose large sums of money. Another is having a drug or alcohol habit. Both require constant feeding and soon can deplete a person's reserves. When this happens, they often resort to unhealthy, even dangerous, actions to acquire money to feed their habit.

Look around in your life and see the little things you may be doing that are depleting you in increments. Unhealthy snacks, even an unhealthy diet, slowly deplete your health, your vitality, and life span. It almost guarantees you will have a debilitating disease down the road. Five-dollar coffee is another example of excessive spending needlessly. Constantly buying expensive items declaring that you have "made it" oftentimes leads to wasteful spending. Some will do this even when they can't afford it.

Listening

This ability can often be compromised. It happens when someone tells you about a way to get rich quick, like betting on a horse, buying a certain stock or an item that is sure to grow in value in a very short time span. There are many get-rich-quick schemes out there. The one who gets rich is the one selling/promoting them. They stimulate your desire to have more. You get excited about the prospect and jump in. Only later, after you have spent your money, time, and energy trying to make it happen do you realize that getting involved was not in your best interest. This is a great time to listen to the small guiding voice from within when it recommends caution before moving forward.

Thinking

Knowing that you have a tendency to deplete your resources, your energy levels, and your health, you must take the time to think deeply upon what you are entering into when a new situation is presented. Will this situation feed you or leave you depleted, undermined, and without resources? Doing this deep level of examination will be the best way to get at the root of the concept and understand all the myriad ways it works. The goal of the concept and its patterns is to undermine you and keep you from having what resources you need to move forward and grow with personal power and strength. Another aspect of thinking is seeking to discover the concept that uses this pattern as a means of maintaining access to "the doorway home."

Program

I am becoming aware of depleting habits. I am controlling my spending. I am minimizing my indulgences. I am no longer indulging in wasteful things. I am thinking twice before I buy or invest.

How does this pattern play out in the various Selves?

Emotional Self

Do you get easily worked up?

Do you frequently feel emotionally spent?

Do you cause others to become depleted?

Physical Self

Do you overindulge?

Do you spend without saving?

Do you tax others with labor?

Material Self

Do you indulge in costly habits/hobbies?

Do you buy cheap goods?

Do you fail to take care of your possessions?

Do you damage the property of others?

Social Self

Are you always on the go?

Always mixing socially?

Do you participate in excessive entertaining?

Are you overly demanding of friends?

Spiritual Self

Do you sacrifice too much of yourself?

Do you engage in excessive volunteering?

Do you make charitable contributions to the detriment of your budget?

Are you overly devout?

DESPERATION

This is a pattern that is interwoven with others, such as laziness, denial, sacrifice, and depletion. Any one of those patterns can lead to desperation and exhaust the resources of a person on every level, thus creating feelings of desperation. Desperation occurs when the person feels that they are at their wits end. They do not see, nor can they think of, a way out of their situation. This feeling can sometimes lead to the committing of a crime or, even worse, suicide.

Seeing

In all patterns of behavior, your mind gives you signs that the pattern is about to begin. Your mind will continue to talk to you through the entire flow of the pattern's life cycle, right up to fulfillment of the expectation associated with the pattern. This is done so that you have a chance to change the outcome of the pattern and create a new and improved you.

If you don't see the signs, such as a dwindling bank account, negative feedback from your employer from a decrease in sales, and distance in your relationships (to name a few), then you do not have a chance to stop its progression. Learn to have eyes that see and ears that hear. A Universal Teaching for desperation is found in Matthew 13:15–16: "For this people's heart is waxed gross, and their ears are dull of listening, and their eyes they have closed; lest at any time they should see with their eyes, and hear with their ears, and should understand with their heart, and should be converted, and I should heal them. But blessed are your eyes, for they see; and your ears, for they hear."

Listening

This is also a very important part of gaining control over this detrimental pattern. In all listening applications, it is vital to hear what you say to yourself, and especially to others. You may harden your tone and choice of words, which leads to sounding like an attack. You may also cry for help. However, you may not directly ask for any number of reasons, which will be ego-based. Examples include: "I don't want anyone to think I am weak." "I can't control this or that." "I don't trust anyone. I will not open myself up."

Outside input can also trigger the pattern. Statements such as, "You better do this." This could lead you to losing your resources and place you in a situation of desperation. Another example: "You need to put your money in this stock or that bond." You may also get caught up in a get-rich-quick scheme and lose what you have. Obviously, you need to be mindful and investigate before acting. Also, question why the end goal of the transaction is being presented to you. Just keep in mind if your need is to end up in a state of desperation, and you make no effort to stop and question it, then you will continue on that path.

Thinking

Here, like in all patterns, you must spend time pondering how this pattern works in your life. You need to employ these Universal Teachings: "Look back in order to see ahead." and "That which hath been is now; and that which is to be hath already been" (Ecclesiastes 3:15). Think back to any situation where you felt desperate. What type of situation was it? How many similar situations have you experienced that facilitated that emotional feeling? It has happened in the past. Your personal history does repeat. Read Universal Teaching again from Ecclesiastes 3:15. Because of the time and place, each episode may look different; however, the same circumstances and energy are at work. Now also think about how you resolved the situation. How did you get through it? What were the actions you took?

Program
I am becoming aware of my patterns. I am not receptive to desperation.
I am never in a situation I cannot master.

How does this pattern play out in the various Selves?
Emotional Self
What do you think you are missing?
What are you willing to do to get what you think you need?
Why do you think you need it?
Physical Self
What are you willing to do to achieve your goal?
Why do you think you need it?
Material Self
What are you willing to sacrifice to get what you want?
What are you willing to do to get what you want?
Why do you think you need it?
Applicable Universal Teaching: "For what is a man profited, if he shall gain the whole world, and lose his own soul?" (Matthew 16:26).
Social Self
Are you desperate to be accepted by others?
What are you willing to do to be accepted by others?
Why do you think you need the acceptance of others?
Reflect on Lao Tzu's directive: "Care about what other people think and you will always be their prisoner."

Spiritual Self
Do you want God/Jesus/Buddha/Shiva/Ganesh to handle what is going on instead of doing your part?

Why do you think you need them to do it for you?

Meditate on this scripture from Genesis 1:26: "And God said, Let us make man in our image, after our likeness; and let them have dominion over the fish of the sea, and over the fowl of the air, and over the cattle, and over all the earth, and over every creeping thing that creepeth upon the earth."

DISAPPOINTMENT

This is another offshoot of perfectionism with its own basis for expression. Disappointment is often the result of unfulfilled expectations. The expectations may be based on what you or another person should have or could have done in a particular situation. Because you had a particular expectation as to how things should have unfolded, and they didn't go the way you anticipated, the disappointment sets in.

Seeing

Since history repeats itself, you need to be aware when your expectations of a situation are forming. As an example, say you are invited to a gathering, and you begin to think about who is going to be there and what you are going to do together. The person may or may not show up. This would result in disappointment because all of your planning and imagining of what was going to unfold never materializes. When you start thinking, planning, and daydreaming about tomorrow, that is when you need to stop and examine what is going on and where you are in the cycle of disappointment. Thinking, planning, and daydreaming about tomorrow is a setup. You are setting the stage for the disappointment to manifest. In almost every pattern, you set the stage for it to occur based on what your particular need is. In other words, which concepts and patterns have been stimulated?

Listening

This is another one of those "two voices talking" situations. One voice is inside your head. The other voice is what others say. As I mentioned earlier, you hear what you want to hear. This implies that you must seek to understand what is really being said versus what you want to be said. Words, when taken the wrong way, could stimulate a chain of events in your mind that are unfounded and not achievable. You may think they said one thing when in fact they said another thing, which had a completely different intent.

Thinking

In order to avoid disappointment, you must think clearly about what is unfolding. Remind yourself that this has this occurred in the past, although the current look of it is different —because of the time that has elapsed, the environment, and the players. The point here is the energy is the same even though it looks entirely different. Learning to see and recall (look back in order to see ahead) the last time this happened will give you the opportunity to avoid the outcome of disappointment. Another aspect of thinking is seeking to discover the concept that uses this pattern as a means of maintaining access to "the doorway home."

Program

I am avoiding disappointment. I am aware of my need to be disappointed.
I am controlling my unrealistic expectations. I am grounded in my planning so as to avoid disappointments.

How does this pattern play out in the various Selves?
Emotional Self

What types of situations and/or events create disappointments?
In what ways do you set the stage for disappointment?
Do you have unattainable expectations of others?
Who disappoints you and why?
Do others fail to live up to your expectations?
Remember: disappointment can lead to anger and disease.

Physical Self

In what ways/areas are you disappointed in yourself? Why?
When you become disappointed, what do you do?
Do you indulge in comfort foods, then feel guilty for doing so?
Do you find yourself in vicious cycles?

Material Self

What types of situations create disappointment?
Are you disappointed in any of your relationships?
Are you disappointed in your kids or other family members?
Are you disappointed in your job?
Are you disappointed in your earnings?

Are you disappointed in the way you have to live?

Social Self

What types of situations create disappointment?

Are you disappointed in your social life? In what ways?

Are you disappointed in your friends? In what ways?

Spiritual Self

What type of situations create disappointment? In what ways?

Are you disappointed in your religion? In what ways?

Are you disappointed in your spiritual leaders? In what ways?

DISSATISFACTION

This is another one of those obvious patterns. However, there are subtleties to be aware of because they are harder to spot. As one becomes aware, they develop the ability to see the pattern at work on all levels. Like the patten of perfectionism and disappointment, as well as the others mentioned above, nothing is ever good enough, never done right . . . nothing is perfect! Not the relationship, the kids, the workplace, or coworkers. Some examples of this patten at work is the need to move every now and then because of some made-up reason. There is always a rational, justifiable reason behind the dissatisfaction in their mind though. The same applies to a car. It may need to be replaced every three or four years. "I've grown tired of it" is often heard in the expression of this pattern. This is a very costly pattern of behavior. It ties into the pattern of depletion, which can lead to denial.

Seeing

Here, a perception is developed to see what is not in keeping with the person's expectations as to how it should be. Something is always not right. Always! Learn to recognize what you see that stimulates your thoughts of dissatisfaction. There are specific things you see that that trigger the pattern. Make a note of these and add them to your dictionary so that when they appear, you will know that dissatisfaction is at work.
As an example, say you go out to dinner. The service is slow, your food is bland, or it's not what you expected it to taste like. You are displeased with everything. On the surface, you are justified in your feelings. However, there are other energies that have played into this experience. Those aside, it would be wise to question what other forms of dissatisfaction are at work in your life. Remember, everything happens for a reason, even when you cannot see, hear, or understand why. This is also why questioning what is going

on within is so vital in becoming aware and in becoming the new you. Every pattern seeks and finds a way to fulfill its expectation, validating the concept as true.

Listening

This is one of those patterns where the listening is all about what you say. You need to learn to hear what you say to yourself and to others. After all, the pattern affects your relationship with others. You may attack others out of being dissatisfied with them, what they are doing, or how they are acting or speaking.

Thinking

One must incorporate the seeing and listening aspects into their thinking. Why is it that something stimulates dissatisfaction? Where does the dissatisfaction come from? Who are you emulating? Is this a consistent thing? In every aspect of thinking throughout this work, because whatever concept and pattern of behavior you're manifesting is coming from somewhere. Maybe you've seen it in action before. It may be that someone is always voicing it. Maybe it's just an attitude that you feel coming from someone. Sometimes a look, an energy can say many things. A picture of someone's face can even say a thousand words.

   In the examples presented, you've seen the attitude of dissatisfaction demonstrated. Now you are incorporating it in your life because you found that it does validate the concept as being true. So look at it in your seeking. Think about all the different ways in which you become dissatisfied. In that way you can understand where it's coming from. Once understood, you can resolve that issue and begin to move forward and get the element and energy of dissatisfaction out of your life. Another aspect of thinking is seeking to discover the concept that uses this pattern as a means of maintaining access to "the doorway home."

Program

I am aware when dissatisfaction is at work. I am becoming more accepting of others. I am becoming more patient with others. I am eliminating dissatisfaction from my life.

How does this pattern play out in the various Selves?
Emotional Self.

What are all the things others do to stimulate dissatisfaction?

In what ways are you dissatisfied with yourself? With members of your family?

Physical Self

In what area of Self are you dissatisfied?

How does that make you feel?

What are you doing to fix it?

Material Self

Are you dissatisfied with your life? Why?

Are you dissatisfied with your relationships? Why?

Are you dissatisfied with your work? Why?

Are you dissatisfied with your income? Why?

Are you dissatisfied with your home? Why?

Are you dissatisfied with your car? Why?

What type of situation stimulates satisfaction in you?

Social Self

What types of situations create dissatisfaction? Are you dissatisfied with your social standing? Why? Are you dissatisfied with your friends? Why?

What personalities stimulate dissatisfaction?

Are you outgoing? The center of attention? An introvert?

Spiritual Self

In what ways are you spiritually dissatisfied? With your religion? Your place of worship? The minister? The people in the congregation?

DISTRACTION

The pattern of distraction ties into some of the other patterns. It can be used in the success and failure pattern as well as the depletion pattern, always being late pattern, and the procrastination pattern. With distraction, the person's attention is easily captured by the "new, shiny object." In doing so, whatever they were working on, or needed to work on, takes a back seat. Now their attention is focused on the new thing. This pattern does a lot of damage because it detracts from what is essential to move forward. Moving forward allows you to complete projects, fulfill commitments, enhance relationships, and grow and develop as a person.

Seeing

This is an important aspect of getting this pattern under control. When a person has this pattern, there are many things that can easily catch their attention. It may start as a fleeting glance, and then you think, Oh I should take care of that before I go. That one thought sets the stage for incompletion, being late to attend a function, or not turning in a project. One must become attuned to when they are indulging in distraction.

Listening

This is another one of those patterns where the two voices speak to you. One says, "You can deal with that later." The other says, "Let's take care of that now." There is also the input from others. Someone may ask you to do this or that before you go, or before you start on the next project. It may come in the form of a personal favor, a request, or even a demand. Depending on who it comes from will determine how you respond. Keep in mind that if you have a tendency to be distracted, you will always be aware of opportunities to become so. This is why it is a pattern of behavior. People develop this to avoid reaching and manifesting their power. In building personal power, they may lose the access to "the doorway back home," the spiritual plane of peace and harmony.

Thinking

The questions here are, "Why do I get easily distracted?" "What purpose does it serve?" "Who did I learn this from?" and "Why have I developed this pattern?" It is essential in all matters relating to Self to question the whys and wherefores. Through questioning, insights are achieved. These insights lead to understandings. Understandings lead to control. Control leads to mastery.

Program

I am controlling the tendency to be distracted. I am staying focused on my tasks at hand. I am completing my assignments on time.

How does this pattern play out in the various Selves?
Emotional Self
In what ways do you distract yourself?
Do you distract others from their tasks?
Physical Self
What types of distractions do you employ to keep yourself from getting healthier?
Why do you let that happen?
How does this fit into your concept of competition?
Material Self

In what ways do you allow distraction to lead you to incompletions and denial? Why?

How does this affect your personal relationships with others?

Social Self

How does this pattern affect your social life?

Are you always late to dinners and social get-togethers?

How does this behavior affect your friends?

Spiritual Self

Do distractions keep you from attending spiritual practices or services?

EMBELLISHING

This pattern is like lying, but different. Here, the person starts out with a truth, a real experience. However, in the telling there are more aspects than actually occurred. It does not matter the experience, or emotional relationship. In either case, it was more wonderful or horrible than experienced. The need to be more, or to seek pity, is present. The greatest example is that of a fisherman and his catch. When he tells the story of the "one that got away," it is always a monster-sized fish. This is where eight inches equals a foot and half.

Seeing

This is hard to see, especially in oneself; however, within the self the person knows they are making a story to be greater than the actual events. In others, it is harder to know the truth until you know the other person. At that level of understanding, you know when a mountain has just been made out of a molehill. Usually, the embellishing of a story comes with enthusiasm in order to make it appear true.

Listening

This is where really paying attention to what is being said and what is being implied is important. There is usually an intent behind the exaggeration. It could be for manipulation purposes. It is also possible that the person's mind would tell them not to embellish because it is not necessary. However, those who have this pattern make it an embedded habit that is hard to break. It takes a conscious effort to control one's speech before it is uttered.

Thinking

This is where the control really begins. If you know that this is something you do, then it is easier to stop doing it with effort and understanding the need, the motivation. I had a cousin who was constantly telling stories of his exploits. Some were true and exaggerated; others were outright lies. When we would be around people, he would always say to me, "Wasn't that true?" I had no choice but to answer yes. After all, he was my cousin, and I did not want to embarrass him. I also knew that the people we were with knew him and well enough to know when his stores were true and magnified, and when he was lying. Ahh, the follies of youth.

Program
I am truthful in all situations. I am never seeking to manipulate others. I am not seeking to impress others. I am comfortable being who I am. I am improving my life.

How does this pattern play out in the various Selves?
Emotional Self
In what ways do you exaggerate your accomplishments?
Who do you try to impress with embellished stories?
Physical Self
What do you do with your appearance that is an exaggeration? Why?
How does this fit in to your concept of competition?
Material Self
Do you present to the world more than you really have? Why?
How does this affect your personal relationships with others?
Social Self
Is exaggeration a technique you use in social settings, especially when you feel less than others?
How does exaggerating affect your friends?
Spiritual Self
Do you present a false pious persona to others?

EXCESS

"There's no such thing as too much." This was once told to me by a former boss who was one of the many unhappy wealthy people I've met. He disowned his kids, divorced, and left an $800 million dollar estate in trust to his current paramour when he died, leaving nothing for his daughter, the only serving child. People who chase after money and think it will bring happiness are fooling themselves. Yes, it brings comfort, and sometimes the "respect and adulation" of others. As for peace and happiness, not necessarily. This is a pattern that is difficult to satiate. It pursues whatever the person's need, want, or desire might be. But they can never get enough of it. This pattern can also be tied into and lead to patterns such as depletion, self-destruction, and desperation. Here are a few Universal Teachings about this need to have more and more.

"Whoever loves money never has money enough;
whoever loves wealth is never satisfied with his income.
This too is meaningless."
—Ecclesiastes 5:10

"A stingy man is eager to get rich and is unaware
that poverty awaits him."
—Proverbs 28:22

"And again I say unto you, It is easier for a camel to go through the eye of a needle,
than for a rich man to enter into the Kingdom of God."
—Matthew 19:24

"Contentment is the greatest wealth."
—Buddha

"In a country well governed, poverty
is something to be ashamed of.
In a country badly governed,
wealth is something to be ashamed of."
—Confucius

Seeing

With this pattern, is easy enough for the person to see when they are indulging. Unfortunately, that doesn't mean they will stop in their pursuit. There are so many stories of people who, using drugs or alcohol as examples, have lost everything because of their desire to get more. Yes, these are really addictions; however, the pattern is the same, in essence. Here is a different kind of example: A friend of mine who owned a bar and a home began with buying liquor novelty decanters online. He bought around 700 of them. They are still in a storage unit, and he pays a$100 a month to house them. Then he moved into buying cars. Some are junkers, and some are rather unique, like an ambulance that he kept parked outside his bar.

Needless to say, he went through all of his money, lost the bar, and had to sell his home. Today, he lives on Social Security and is a mystery shopper in a rundown mobile home. Another example centers around hoarders: They hold on to everything, and some go collecting and gathering what they see on the side of the road. The Universal Teaching applicable to this pattern is: "Excess leads to rejection."

Listening

The pattern of excess is more about internal communication than external. A friend may be the external voice and say: "You already have that." "Where you going to put that?" "What do you need that for? Are you crazy?" Your internal voice will talk to you on two levels: "Go for it!" and "What do you think you are going to do with that?" When you hear either of these comments, know the pattern of excess is at work.

Thinking

This pattern requires questioning before an action is taken. You have to think about the internal communication and ponder the questions your mind asks you. In this situation, there are two minds talking: your true spiritual mind and your ego. It is the ego that is the main source of the trouble. The ego is insecure and requires the abundance of whatever you think you need, want, or desire.

Program

I am not holding on to useless things. I am living within my means. I am living in balance with my true needs. I am controlling my wants and desires.

How does this pattern play out in the various Selves?
Emotional Self

In what ways are you excessive?

Do you crave attention from your partner?

From your children?

From others?

What do you expect from others?

Physical Self

Do you overindulge in:

Alcohol?

Sex?

Drugs?

Partying?

Overexercising?

Overworking?

Material Self

Do you overeat?

Do you have more possessions than you need?

Do you keep acquiring more things?

Social Self

Do you have to be with people all the time?

Do you feel obligated to entertain?

Do you expect others to spend time with you?

Do you expect others to entertain you?

Spiritual Self

Are you overly religious?

Do you attend your place of worship multiple times a week?

Are you strict with yourself and your family?

What do you expect from others?

FEAR & DOUBT

This pattern, I believe, affects everyone to some degree or another. Some use bravado to hide their fear; others live with it; others seek to understand its roots and how to eliminate fear and doubt from the actions and reactions in their life.

Seeing

The energy of fear and doubt is difficult to see. Nonetheless, your mind will give you signs that you are entering into a cycle of fear and doubt in a relationship. You may see something that will trigger a thought that you can relate to that stimulates doubt or fear. Here's my personal example: As a kid, I was attacked by a black Cocker Spaniel.

Whenever I see that type of dog, I know I am experiencing doubt and fear. I immediately ask myself, "What am I currently involved in regarding my life, and how will that energy undermine me?" and "Where am I headed that I am uncertain about?" and "What is going on in my life right now that is causing me doubt?"

All of those thoughts are stimulated by seeing a black Cocker Spaniel. Those thoughts tell me to question what is going on and to make an attitude adjustment. Changing an attitude can often change the outcome of a situation. It may also require gaining more information and knowledge about what I am doing and where I am going. Think about all the signs and symbols that represent doubt and fear that you have experienced in the past. They will replay until you eliminate the doubt associated with that particular sign.

Listening

If you pay attention to what you are hearing, your internal voice will work for you or against you. It may tell you to stop doing what you are doing, or to keep going. The difficult part is knowing which voice is right. To keep going could take you past your doubt and lead you to success. The other is building on your fears. The core issue here is which concept, need, want, or desire is being pursued. There is also the possibility that someone will say something to you to stimulate that doubt or fear in your ability to handle a situation or project.

Thinking

In all matters, thinking is an essential element. Here, you must listen to your thoughts. What line of thinking are you using? The one that validates the doubt and fear, or the one that wants you to fight it and move forward? Another aspect of thinking is seeking to discover the concept that uses this pattern as a means of maintaining access to "the doorway home." Thinking is a tool to help you master, in all situations, whatever you are confronting.

Program

The programs here center on building courage and confidence.

I am mastering this current project. I am gaining control over my fears. I am never placed in a situation I cannot overcome.

How does this pattern play out in the various Selves?

Emotional Self

We all have doubts and fears. Fear of dying is one of the strongest because we don't know what to expect. What are your doubts, fears, and phobias? In what areas of your life do they show up? What is the root source of your fears? Who in your immediate family has similar fears?

Physical Self

Are you afraid of getting hurt? How has your fear stopped you from physical activities? Are you afraid you are not strong enough? Are you afraid you are not athletic enough?

Material Self

Do you doubt you have the ability, the knowledge, or the credentials to earn a good living? To support a family? Are you afraid of being broke? Becoming homeless?

Social Self

Do you feel not smart enough?

Do you feel like you don't fit in?

Do you fear rejection? Or not being invited? Or not being liked?

Spiritual Self

Do you fear you are not religious enough?

Are you doubting if you are a good person?

Do you fear not going to heaven because of something you have done?

GUILT

This pattern—along with anger, resentment and frustration—is another form of emotional energy that, when internalized, can cause ill health. Guilt, as a pattern, is often employed to gain control and dominance over another. Parents guilt their children. Sometimes teachers guilt their students. The church guilts its followers. Instilling guilt in a person is based in fear. The guilt pattern has a specific message: If you do not follow the dictates of your parents, your teachers, or the church, then you will be punished. The dictates are the rules and regulations established by each entity to keep you in line.

Keeping people in line and creating order and rules is not necessarily a bad thing. As a society, we do need rules and regulations to maintain balance, harmony, and cooperation to successfully grow and build communities and families. The problem arises when you want to do something that the ruling party feels is wrong. And when you do it, for whatever rational, logical, and justifiable reason, you are guilty of breaking a rule and stepping over the line; therefore you need to be punished. Guilt is also a form of self-punishment, except it is internalized. Like cancer, guilt can eat at you and be all-consuming.

Seeing

If you look around at what life presents you, you'll see opportunities for guilt everywhere. Christian Universal Teachings are often not followed by the masses of Christians. This teaching is relevant to striving for unity instead of guilt: "That ye love one another; as I have loved you, that ye also love one another. By this shall all men know that ye are my disciples, if ye have love one to another" (John 13:34–35). In people's minds, there are rational, logical, and justifiable reasons not to offer love, assistance, money, time, and effort. Here are a few prime examples. We all see the beggars on the street corners. Very few people give them anything. We see people, especially a woman or two young girls, broke down on the side of the road, and cars whiz by. We disdainfully see homeless people living in cardboard boxes under bridges. When you see any of the examples above, do you give aid in any form? If not, does that bother you? If it does, that is guilt at work. Some do give. They support the shelters and food distribution services. However, far too few remain involved in a long-term and truly beneficial way. The cash-rich are blinded by their need for more. It seems the following Universal Teaching is applicable to this situation:

> "No servant can serve two masters;
> for either he will hate the one, and love the other;
> or else he will hold to the one, and despise the other.
> Ye cannot serve God and Mammon."
> —Luke 16:13

Listening

Oftentimes, we hear things said to us directly, or in a religious service, that imply we are not doing enough of this or that. "You don't help around the house! You don't take care of the kids. Did you call your brother? Why don't you call him more often?" These remarks are from family and friends. Work provides another source of guilt. "Where's the project you were assigned? Why are you late with that report?" All of these are stimulants for the pattern of guilt to manifest.

Thinking

Here, you are more likely to get sidetracked for thinking in a guilt-infused way. You feel guilty because you were told that you are wrong. That the thoughts you generate, or dwell upon, are even sinful. Questions arise: "Why do I want to do this?" "What am I trying to accomplish?" "What am I trying to fulfill?" "Is it a need, want, or desire? If so, where do those feelings come from?"

Here is a different perspective on sin, which you may not agree with, but at least ponder this explanation: Even if it involves killing another human being, the principle is the same. A sin is something a person does that society, the church, family systems, and the culture deem sinful. The reason the person does what they do is because they are trying to satisfy a need within. That is not to say that the need is justified, but from a patternistic perspective, the person feels that it is.

Here is an example: A sadist is walking up the street and says, "If only I could beat up someone. That would make me feel so much better." On the other side of the street, a masochist is walking in the opposite direction. The masochist crosses the road at the same time the sadist does, and they bump into each other and the conflict unfolds. Both parties received what they were asking for. The sadist was able to beat someone up, and the masochist was able to get beat up. Satisfaction and fulfillment of their individual patterns was accomplished.

In this example, you can change out the environment, but the outcome and pattern still remain. This is more easily seen between battered wives (masochist) and husbands (sadist). What's even more telling is that each party swears they will never be in an abusive situation again. However, the masochist will either go back to their spouse or find a new abuser, even if it's at work. The need, the concept, and its pattern is to "be abused." It may be physical, verbal, or emotional. Abuse is a way to control another person.

Program

I am a worthy person. I am not allowing myself to be abused. I am not allowing others to take advantage of me. I am being more helpful to those in need.

How does this pattern play out in the various Selves?

Emotional Self

Do you forget celebratory events?

Do you say hurtful things?

Do you neglect the Physical Self?

Do you not carefully observe your diet?

Do you have physical disciplines?

Material Self

Do you squander money and resources?

Social Self

Are you late, rude, and thoughtless?

Spiritual Self

Are you an unbeliever?

Do you refuse to attend church?

IMPATIENCE

This pattern of behavior has elements of inconsideration of others, rudeness by always interrupting, and dissatisfaction with how long something is taking to be accomplished. This is almost always directed outside of Self. It is always someone else's fault that things are not going as fast as you wished they would.

Seeing

A perfect example of the impatience pattern is waiting for your order to be delivered, especially at a restaurant. It could be the food, drinks, or a package that was shipped and has not arrived. This pattern applies to anything else you are waiting on. When you feel yourself getting antsy, know that the pattern of impatience is at work.

Listening

Here, the examples are easy to see and hear. When you are listening to someone speak and you feel the urge to add your perspective or understanding to the conversation, know right then and there that the pattern is beginning to unfold. When you hear yourself interrupting what someone else is saying, recognize that you are being impatient. The pattern is at work. Yes, you will have an easy explanation for butting in: "My mind works too fast." That may be true, but in order to become a better person, one must learn to listen. There may be valuable information coming your way, and if you are always interjecting, you may end up missing crucial guidance. A relevant teaching is, "You have two ears and one mouth." Learn to listen.

Thinking

Every pattern evolves from a concept in the subconscious mind. Some concepts create a few patterns. Each relate to specific stimulus and what might be unfolding. As examples, the patterns of denial, depletion, self-pity, and self-destruction can all stem from the same basic concept, or concepts. They could feel unworthy, undeserving, or inadequate. The thinking here is from whom did you learn this pattern: Mom or Dad? Remember, each of them teaches us different ways of behaving. Knowing who you emulate will go a long way in helping you understand yourself. It will also help you let go of those patterns and their concepts so that you can evolve to a higher consciousness. This would also be a reflection of a better you.

Program

I am patient with myself in everything. I am patient with others.

How does this pattern play out in the various Selves?

Emotional Self

In what ways are you impatient with yourself and others?

Does being impatient set you up for disappointment/anger/frustration/aggression?

Physical Self

Does your impatience create pressure and frustration when goals are not attained in short time periods?

What do you expect of others in regards to timeframes?

Material Self

Are you always in a hurry to get to where you want to go?

Are you impatient in reaching your financial goals?

Social Self

In what situations are you impatient with your friends in social settings?

How does this pattern affect your friends? Your partner?

Spiritual Self

Does this set you up for disappointment?

Do you feel that God, Jesus, Buddha, Shiva, or whomever you call your higher power, is slow to respond, or unresponsive?

How does that make you feel?
What other patterns are triggered by these feelings?

IMPOSITION

The pattern of imposition works in two ways. First, it's activated by feeling imposed upon by others. Second, it's activated by your use of the pattern to impose your needs, wants, or desires on others. This pattern is often experienced with resentment and used in partnership with obligation and manipulation.

Seeing

Like other patterns that we use, it is often difficult to see it operating in ourselves. The subtleties of any pattern often escape our attention, not to mention that we generally think of ourselves as being right and not patternistic. If you examine how you use obligation and or manipulation, it will be easier to see how you use it, as well as how it is used to manipulate and obligate you. The keys will often be the actions and words you use to get your way.

Listening

This is a skill that is hardly ever used by people to hear what they say to others. For some, talking is just their stream of consciousness made verbal. However, for growth it is essential to listen to yourself when you are talking to someone else. In this case, learn to hear the words you use to get your way or to impose your will on another. In the same regard, decipher the words that others use to impose their will upon you.

Thinking

This aspect is more about questioning yourself as to why you feel the need to impose your will on another. Obviously, there is something you want from someone when you act this way. What do they have that you feel or believe you don't have? Also, question why you think you need whatever "it" is. What do you think having "it" will do for you? Question why you are open to being manipulated, obligated, and imposed upon. If it is coming your way, then you drew it to you, so own it. Then begin to understand why so it doesn't keep happening.

Program

I am not open to being imposed upon. I am questioning the motives of others. I am resistant to the will of others. I am in control of my emotions. I am not imposing my will on others.

How does this pattern play out in the various Selves?
Emotional Self
What are the needs, wants, and desires that I am imposing upon others to provide for me?
What are the emotional actions I use to impose upon others?
What do others emote, that I feel, makes me think they are imposing on me?
Why am I susceptible to being imposed upon?
How do I use the energy of imposing on others? What words? What actions?
Physical Self
How does imposition from others affect my health?
Why are there some things, such as certain foods, that are presented to me for my benefit that I feel or think are impositions?
Material Self
How do I impose my will to gain a financial advantage over others?
In the same respect, how is this done to me? How can I attune myself to a healthier frequency to prevent others from imposing on me?
How do I get control over this energy in my business and personal life?
Social Self
What are some social situations that arise where I feel the need to get my way and impose my desire?
How do I go about imposing on others in these gatherings?
What actions do I employ to get my way?
How am I manipulated and imposed upon by others?
What are the signs that this taking place?
Spiritual Self
Do I feel that the family's religion or my spiritual practice is being forced on me?
Why do I feel that way?

LAZINESS
The pattern of laziness has its roots in different concepts. It also works in tandem with other patterns of behavior, such as success and failure, denial, depletion, deprivation, and

procrastination, to mention a few. By looking at the list of associated patterns, it is easy to see this pattern at work.

Seeing

When you see something that requires attention at any level and you say, "I will get to that, but first I need to . . ." That is you putting off what needs to be done now. This, too, is attached to the patten of distraction. Putting off something that needs to be done today sets you up for a serious or costly problem. There is a saying amongst the lazy at heart: "Why do today what you can put off until tomorrow?" I am sure you have heard that said in either truth or jest. Just know that many a statement made in jest is a reflection, on some level, of the truth.

An example of this pattern at work would be someone living in an RV or mobile home, dependent on propane for heat and hot water. Winter is coming, and they know the next few nights are going to be the first chill of the year. In fact, it is broadcast on the news that it will be an "Arctic blast." The person, knowing that this is going to unfold, does not bother to ensure that the tanks are full and instead goes to bed. In the middle of the night the tanks run out of propane, and the person wakes up to a freezing home with no hot water. In the military there is a saying: "Poor planning promotes poor performance." This played out in the example above.

Listening

There are many things heard that require attention—some immediate, some later. Those issues that require immediate attention, when put off for one reason or another, will be the ones that cost you the most. Keep in mind that the lazy mind will have a justifiable, logical, and rational reason for not acting immediately. Here is an example of this. At a trade convention, a business owner is told in casual conversation that the state of California is going after companies that do not list Prop 65 on the products. The owner, in this case, did not pay attention to the statement and therefore took no action to ensure his products were compliant with the law. Long story short: it cost him $35,000 in fines and legal fees.

Thinking

In this realm, the use of justification and rationalization are employed every time a task or chore is presented. Here, there is a difference between procrastination and laziness. Procrastinators will put off doing what needs to be done until tomorrow. Lazy people will simply never do it. They have in their mind a great reason not to. Once again, you can see justification and rationalization taking affect. A perfect example is the husband who does not help with home chores, like washing dishes, cleaning off the table, and folding clothes. After all, he went to work and feels that it is not his job, not his responsibility. Should this pattern be one of yours, then use the understanding that when you come up with a good or great excuse for not participating, laziness is at work.

Program
I am a partner sharing work at home. I am participating in what is presented. I am a helpmate to all. I am energized.

How does this pattern play out in the various Selves?
Emotional Self
Are you unwilling to give?
Are you inconsiderate of others?
Physical Self
Are you a couch potato?
Do you do as little as possible?
Material Self
Do you not make the effort to move forward financially?
Do you do as little as possible at work?
Social Self
Do you minimize being with people?
Is socializing simply too much emotional effort?
Spiritual Self
Do you feel like not bothering with a task because what is the point of it?

LYING
This is another self-serving pattern. It is used for many different purposes: to get what one wants without working for it; to avoid getting in trouble for actions taken that the person knew were wrong. Lying is also part of the tool box of manipulation, demanding,

and taking advantage of others. Sometimes people lie to themselves because they do not want to admit they were wrong.

Seeing

It is easier to see this pattern at work in others when you know the truth, when you know the facts associated with what they are presenting. A person does not see this in themself because they already know they are lying. Lying has become a mentally contrived intent. Lying is used to manifest one's intent without the exercise of will. This is where the manipulation comes into play—having others use their will to bring into being the person's desire.

Listening

Like seeing, it is easier to hear when someone else is doing it. In listening to others it is always prudent to listen carefully and verify what is being said. As President Ronald Regan said, "Trust, but verify."

Thinking

The truth of the matter is the person knows when they are lying and why. They want something. It has nothing to do with needs. It's all about the wants and desires they are unwilling to work for. This pattern is also used to inflate their ego and accomplishments. To overcome this pattern requires effort to control one's conversations. To examine why they have this need. To understand where the fear and doubt lies about one's ability to handle situations and be truly successful.

Program

I am no longer lying to get what I want. I am being honest in every situation.
I am earning respect and admiration through my deeds and actions.

How does this pattern play out in the various Selves?
Emotional Self
In what ways do you lie to yourself about emotional relationships?
Why do you lie to others?
What are you afraid of?
Physical Self

Do you go to the gym and just walk slowly on the treadmill, telling yourself that you are working out?

Do you eat salads only twice a week, if that, and say that you have a good diet? This is lying to yourself as well as others!

Material Self

How does lying manifest in your financial realm?

What false financial images are you presenting?

Social Self

In what ways do you use lying as a social tool?

How does lying affect your social relationships?

Spiritual Self

How are you lying to yourself and others about your spirituality?

What exactly are those lies?

MANIPULATION

This particular pattern is about controlling others. It is designed to get you what you want without any consideration for others' feelings or resources. In fact, one goal of this pattern is to obtain the resources others have by any means. It may be their time, energy, money, or things of a physical nature. This pattern often comes from a doubt in one's ability to achieve on their own. The thought is that they do not have what they need to succeed. Early in life they first learned how to manipulate their parents. From there, the techniques were developed and used on others.

Seeing

The ability to see oneself in action is hard to do. It requires being honest with the Self, another very hard thing to do. However, when you become aware of the desire to have and take what someone else has, it's a sign to you that manipulation is being stimulated. Another scenario is when you feel the need to control a situation or be the manager of every transaction. Through the pattern of manipulation, you stay at the top, at least in your mind. You feel in control.

Listening

When you hear or see resistance to your authority, your mind is making you aware that you are employing the pattern of control. They will say something, either in jest or straightforward: "No! This is not what I want to do." The response will be proportionate to your power over them, their own level of courage and confidence, and how secure they are in the relationship and within themself.

Thinking

When you begin thinking, rationalizing, justifying, and coming up with logical reason as to why you want or need the object of your intent, that is your mind telling you the pattern is being stimulated. This is when you have the opportunity to change your actions, your attitude, and create a new outcome. A new result can reflect the new you.

Program

I am in control of my need to control. I am drawing upon my courage and confidence to achieve my goals, needs, wants, and desires. I am blessed with abundance within.

How does this pattern play out in the various Selves?

Emotional Self

Do you employ manipulation?

Do you manipulate others to get what you want?

In what ways do you allow yourself to be manipulated?

Physical Self

Do you seek to get others to do your work?

Do you manipulate events/situations to avoid work?

Material Self

In what ways do you manipulate to get the best deals?

Social Self

Are you a control freak? Do you seek to be in control?

How do you set things up to go your way?

Spiritual Self

How do you make yourself and others feel guilty?

OBLIGATION

There are two sides to this pattern. One is being obligated to others, and the flip side is making others obligated to you. This pattern, like many others, has setups built in. Here, too, it goes both ways. You set up a situation where another person owes you, and you will also set up a situation that makes you obligated to someone. This pattern can be tied into manipulation in both instances, owing and being owed.

Seeing

Obligation is a hard-to-see pattern until you are in the midst of it. This is more a listening and thinking situation. However, there are signs that will tell you that you are about to set someone up to be obligated to you, or you are being set up to owe someone something. The sign may be meeting an old acquaintance in the supermarket, mall, gym, or simply walking on the beach while on vacation. This is one of the ways your mind works to give you guidance. It will draw to you what you need to see in order to know where you are in the cycle of a pattern.

When this occurs, it is necessary to ask, "When was this person in my life?" "What was going on?" "What was I doing or going through?" Asking these questions will help you understand which particular pattern is at work and where in the flow of it you are. Knowing which pattern is at work, where you are in it, and knowing its previous outcomes will give you an opportunity to change an attitude, action, or behavior, thus changing the outcome to what you want it to be, not what has occurred in the past. This is the opportunity to grow more into the new you.

Listening

There are certain phrases you use to set the stage for an obligatory situation. You are not alone in doing this. Others will, and do, the same to you. It is imperative that you recognize the ones you use and the ones used to snare you. Knowing these and their alternatives will spare you from angst and possible grief and loss. You see, when a person has this pattern, they are highly susceptible to obligation. The biggest area of this occurs in the family. Obviously, parents are at the top of the list. As adult children, we feel obligated to care for our parents. Sometimes in spite of who they were to us. If you have children of your own, there are multiple obligations, most of which are unspoken because it is assumed that, as a parent, you will do the right thing.

Thinking

In this aspect it is essential that you question who and why you are seeking to make another person obligated to you. In the same respect, these questions need to be asked when you think, feel, see, or hear when someone is seeking to make you obligated to them. Remember, this is a learned pattern of behavior. It comes from Mom or Dad. It may even be the exact opposite of them. In either case, it is a way of understanding your own mode of acceptance: approval or rejection.

Program

I am aware of setting the stage to obligate someone. I am aware of being set up. I am aware of being obligated. I am controlling my need to obligate people for my needs. I am in control of my emotions.

How does this pattern play out in the various Selves?

Emotional Self

What are your obligations?

How do you feel about your obligations?

In what ways do make others feel obligated?

Physical Self

Are there physical acts you feel obligated to do?

Do you resent them?

Are there things you obligate others to do?

Material Self

Which obligations do you resent and why?

What do you obligate people to do for you?

Social Self

In what ways do you feel obligated?

Spiritual Self

Are you obligated to go to a house of worship?

OVERCOMPENSATE

This pattern is a setup for emotional turmoil on many levels. A person with this pattern will go out of their way to overcompensate for a wrong they think they may have done to someone. In doing so, they then feel that the other person should reciprocate in some fashion or manner. Therein lies the setup. Now they are expecting something. At the very least, they want a thank-you. When that does not occur, they can become disappointed or angry. Then they feel the urge to attack the person in some form and afterward feel guilty for doing so. To make amends, they overcompensate. Here you can see a vicious cycle unfolding that seems to keep looping back upon itself and at the same time engaging other patterns, such as guilt, resentment, and disappointment.

Seeing

Seeing a subtle pattern at work such as overcompensating is somewhat difficult. Two common signs are constantly doing something for a person or a multitude of people simultaneously; or always buying a little trinket, such as food or a small gift. These are sings of trying to win someone's acceptance, attention, love, and favor. There are certain "shows" that a person may put on to gain your sympathy and make you feel bad about what you have because they do not have it. They want compensation for their lack of having. In some instances, this leads to the other person overcompensating.

Listening

Learning and being attuned to the specific words that trigger this pattern is essential. Just as in seeing something that someone does to trigger you, listening is another avenue. Someone may say something to you that implies you owe them more attention, more time, more money, more favors. This pattern can easily set you up to be manipulated by others who know you have a tendency to overcompensate.

Thinking

This path to understanding cannot be overlooked. Most people do not spend enough time thinking about why they did this or that. Of course, there will be the immediate, logical reason as to why one may have done what they did. If need be, they may even justify the behavior or actions taken. As a final step, they will rationalize the action, saying, "I had no choice." With this pattern, one needs to question from whom did they learn it? What purpose does it serve?

Program

I am aware of when I am overcompensating. I am modifying my behavior.
I am not overcompensating in any area of my life.
I am gaining more control over my emotional responses.

How does this pattern play out in the various Selves?
Emotional Self

In what ways do you overcompensate?
What are the things that cause you to respond in that manner?
Physical Self

What activity do you engage in to prove you are better than someone?

Material Self
In what ways do you seek more more money?

Do you unnecessarily shower people with gifts?

Social Self
Do entertain people excessively?

Are you social every weekend night?

Spiritual Self
Do you go to church, temple, or synagogue every day? Every week?

Do you do good deeds in hopes of being saved?

PERFECTIONISM

Like every other pattern, perfectionism especially detrimental. It creates stress and disharmony with everyone, including Self. This is a pattern of "it's not good enough." You can always see the flaw in others, be it a person or project. The hard part is trying to fix the flaws within them, and especially within yourself. No matter what, it falls short of what you think it should be. This way of seeing things also stimulates the patterns of dissatisfaction, disappointment, intolerance, and rejection. Perfectionism can also stifle, ruin, and create friction in a relationship. In this mindset, no one and nothing is ever good enough.

Seeing
You know when perfectionism is at work because whatever you are working on keeps getting fine-tuned until it is perfect. Of course, there is no way that it can be. However, at some point, you will stop striving, redoing, and looking for the perfect solution. The stopping may be because someone told you to move on and get it done, whatever the project. A perfect example is looking in the mirror as you are ready to go to a dinner, a social gathering, or a performance. You look at and critique yourself and see "perceived flaws." All you notice are the shortcomings in your appearance, your partner's appearance, or your kids' appearances.

Listening
Every pattern has a need and an expectation to be fulfilled. In this pattern, as in many others, your mind is attuned to see and hear those things that tell you there is a flaw. Whenever you begin to see or hear that small voice within—This or that could be better.

If only this or that could be done—you will know that the patten of needing it to be perfect is at work. Perfectionism is a trap in the sense that once you are caught up in it, the seeds of discontent are sown. Other patterns come into play that will lead to stress and eventually to a negative health condition. The Universal Teaching here is: "What is within will manifest without."

Thinking

Every pattern of behavior has its roots in a concept. Every concept tells you how to be in every given situation. The questions here are: "Where does this concept come from? " "Who is it that seeks perfection: Mom or Dad?" "Who is never satisfied with what I have done?" Who told me it could have been better if only I did this or that?" Another aspect of thinking is seeking to discover the concept that uses this pattern as a means of maintaining access to "the doorway home."

Program

I am learning to see the positive in everything. I am becoming more tolerant and accepting. I am in control of my need for perfection. I am producing high-quality work.

How does this pattern play out in the various Selves?
Emotional Self
In what ways do you seek to have the perfect emotional relationship?
In what ways do you seek to have the perfect work relationship?
What do you expect of yourself? What do you expect of your partner?
Physical Self
Do you get frustrated because of your physical appearance?
In what ways are you dissatisfied with Self and others?
Do you strive for the perfect body? What are you doing to accomplish it?
Do you seek to maintain the perfect diet?
Material Self
Do you seek to have the perfect home?
Do you seek to have the perfect car?
Do you seek to have the perfect clothes?
Do you seek to have the perfect job?
Social Self
Do you expect to have the perfect social life?

Do you expect to host perfect social events?

Do you expect to attend perfect events?

Do you expect to have the perfect friends?

What do you demand of yourself in social settings?

What do you demand of your friends?

Spiritual Self

Are you out to be the best? The most pious? What does that mean to you?

What do you think being overly pious will do for you?

Do you expect others to be perfect, whatever their faith may be?

PROCRASTINATION

There are two fundamental reasons for this pattern: doubt and rejection. The doubt comes from a lack of knowledge, skill, or experience. On another level, it comes from a lack of confidence and courage. For some, it is the fear of failing, which is really another way to avoid success. The rejection is one of the end results. It can come about because of being late in delivery of the project or assignment, dealing with a situation, or just plain non-completion. This pattern can be interwoven with other patterns, such as success and failure, always being late, the need for perfection, laziness, and resentment.

Seeing

One way of becoming aware of when this pattern is beginning to go into action is when the person realizes they are being distracted. This, too, is another pattern of behavior. It becomes the method for being late in delivery of the required attention, resources, or project. Becoming aware is essential.

Another insight is being unprepared and not having what is necessary to do the project. Or waiting till the last minute to get what is required. This sets you up for rejection. Here is an example: A trade show is coming up. Marketing and sales material needs to be completed by a certain date in order to be included in the shipment. The person responsible, for one reason or another, does not meet the deadline, and the printed material has to be sent out next-day air to the person attending the show. The material has to be delivered to their hotel and then carried to the show floor. This one transaction triggered feelings of resentment toward the graphics person. This transaction was one of many that would, and did, lead to the termination of the employee, thus the rejection they were seeking was fulfilled.

Listening

This is one of those two minds speaking to the person. One is saying "You need to get this done on time." The other says, "Not to worry! There's plenty of time." The person also becomes attuned to listening for opportunities to get distracted from the task at hand. They may even volunteer to participate in an endeavor or project that is outside their realm just to avoid getting started on their own project.

Thinking

In order for one to grow and move forward in life, pondering the whys and wherefores is essential. Questioning here centers on "Why am I seeking rejection?" Along with it comes, "Where else in my life am I delaying getting involved, or failing to complete or commit to something?" Seek to become aware of all the little and subtle things that distract you. The thoughts that tell you you're not prepared. That you have time to get it done. That it is beyond your capabilities. These are just some of the rationalizations that will be employed.

Program

I am mindful of time. I am getting projects done on schedule. I am not getting distracted. I am gathering what I need to be successful.

How does this pattern play out in the various Selves?

Emotional Self

What are the things you procrastinate about?

How does this impede your moving forward?

How does this affect your partner, family, and friends?

Physical Self

How has this pattern affected your health?

Has it affected the health of others close to you?

Material Self

Has this attitude cost you money and opportunities for growth and advancement?

Social Self

Does this pattern cause you to create a negative energy amongst others with whom you interact?

Do others exclude you from events?

Spiritual Self

Does this behavior prevent you from committing?

Does this behavior prevent you from seeking a greater, deeper understanding of your spiritual life?

REJECTION

Of all the patterns, rejection (and approval), are the foundational modes of expression. In this pattern, the individual seeks rejection in every relationship, both personal and professional. The need for rejection is strong. It is tied into the need for acceptance from Mom. This was presented in the section titled "The Doorway Home."

Seeing

There are so many signs of rejection at work that if one's eyes are open, and awareness to control and change is present, it is hard to miss. Examples include: not participating at home when asked to do something; not doing or finishing necessary projects for home or work; turning in projects and assignments late; forgetting birthdays and anniversaries; ignoring special occasions. Another common example is getting easily distracted into another task. Distraction allows for a logical, rational, and justifiable reason as to why the person was late in doing what had to be done, or why they did not do it at all. There are more examples; in fact, you could probably think of some yourself.

Listening

Signs of the pattern of rejection at work are when someone (a partner, manager, or friend) tells you, "You're late with . . ." Another could be, "You forgot to get . . ." or "Why did you do that?" or "Why did you say that?" Or the opposite: "Why didn't you . . . ?" The list can go on and on. The internal Self will have two voices talking to you. The spiritual voice says, "You need to get this done!" The ego voice says, "You've got time." Or "Did you see that? Let's look at that," or "Let's do that and we will get back to the project shortly." Of course, there will be other statements with the same end result: procrastination and failure to complete.

Thinking

Rejection can tie into every other pattern because it is a foundational issue that must be understood. The workings of this mode of being are so subtle, so be ready to be challenged to see it, hear, it and react to it if this is your modus operandi. In the deepest part of your subconscious mind, right above your Spiritual Self, this mode of expression exists. Remember, this is necessary in your mind to return to the peace and tranquilly of the spiritual dominion where you came from.

Program

I am becoming aware of how rejection operates in my life. I am controlling becoming distracted. I am strengthening my completion of projects and tasks. I am becoming more loving. I am participating more in everything.

How does this pattern play out in the various Selves?

Emotional Self

Do you attack yourself? Do you denigrate yourself? Do you make jokes about yourself? What do you do to cause others to attack you?

Physical Self

Do you find yourself in accidents more than most?

Do you hurt yourself?

Do you cut yourself?

Do you fight with yourself?

Do you feel that death is the ultimate form of rejection?

Material Self

How do you reject opportunities for growth? For financial advancement?

For getting fired?

What types of situations do you create?

What are the logical, rational, justifiable reasons for creating what you do when it is negative?

Social Self

Do you behave inappropriately? Do you use inappropriate language?

Do you display a lack of respect for others?

Do you lack common courtesies?

Do you frequently interrupt other people?

Do you have questionable habits?

Spiritual Self

Do you turn away from your family's religion?

Do you turn away from the belief in God?

Do you reject your spiritual gifts?

RESENTMENT

Life presents many opportunities to express yourself. There are things that can lead one to feel justified in their resentment within in their marriage, family, workplace, and in everyday living and interacting with others. Sometimes you may not even realize that the pattern is at work until something occurs that makes it obvious, such as losing your temper over a situation, person, or event. This is one of those patterns that leads to illness. Resentment can, and often does, lead to anger. Anger is an emotion that eats at you until you let it loose and vent! At that point, things may be said to the person you are angry at that can never be taken back. Those statements may be so hurtful, so detrimental, that the relationship can never be repaired.

Seeing

The subtleties of the pattern of resentment are many. When you notice that a person is living in a way that you wished you could, then know that resentment is at work. You may wonder how they did it. Why do they have what they have? They may not have worked hard for it. It may appear that it was given to them. When you find yourself being jealous of what they have, you may be exercising resentment. When someone does something that affects you or someone else in a negative way, you may resent them for doing what they did. The same holds true for what they may say to you or another. A great example is creating and giving something to someone where you put a lot of effort into the project, the endeavor. They, in turn, reciprocate the gesture with "giveaways," by offering you items they have laying around from their business. You get upset because for them it was an obligatory response with no real feeling behind it. It wasn't anything that required thought or effort!

Listening

In this aspect of the resentment pattern, it is something that is said directly (to you specifically) while you are trying to focus on another dialogue (such as a movie) in a situation. When the voices interfere with you listening to what is being said onscreen, it can stimulate feelings of resentment. The same thing may happen at home. Sometimes even more so. An example of how this triggers resentment and anger is when, if you talk while your friend is listening to news and they tell you to be quiet—with an attitude and energy of anger for interrupting their listening—yet they do to you what they have given you a scolding for. That will set the energy of resentment into motion. You can't do it to them, but they can do it to you!

Thinking

Mindfulness is a key because of the possible internal damage resentment can cause. This pattern demands awareness about the triggers that get you going. Thoughts need to be examined and understood on two levels. The first being, why? Why does what they say or do make you feel resentful? The second question, and just as enlightening, is where does that annoyance come from? Is it Mom? Is it Dad? Or do you operate and strive to be different. As an example, Mom or Dad may be very tolerant of others—not jealous or envious of what others have. They may be complacent with where they are on every level. You, on the other hand, may want more. Much more! Seeing what others have and realizing that your parents didn't strive to have more may be part of the root of this pattern.

Program

I am aware of when resentment is at work. I am letting go of my resentments. I can achieve whatever I set my mind to do, have, or accomplish.

How does this pattern play out in the various Selves?

Emotional Self

What are the things you resent about yourself?

What are the things you resent about others?

Who do you resent and why?

Remember: resentment causes disease.

Physical Self

Do you have a deformity?

Do you have a limitation of sorts?

Do you like the way your body looks?

Do you like the way your body responds to exercise?

Do you like the way your body responds to life?

Material Self

Do you resent being born poor?

Do you resent always struggling to make a living?

Do you resent not being able to live comfortably?

Do you feel you lack money?

Social Self

Do you find yourself lacking friends?

Do you feel you don't have what it takes to keep up?

Do you resent the expectations put upon you to act or respond in a particular way?

What are the things you resent about being social?

Spiritual Self

Were you raised in a way that forced beliefs and principles on you?

Were you made to participate in rituals?

Are you resentful of not getting your prayers answered?

What are the things you resent about your religious obligations?

SACRIFICE

This pattern often has its roots in the concepts presented to the Spiritual Self. Thinking and doing for others is a virtue. And on some levels those statements are true. However, there is a limit when that should be curtailed. Here is a Universal Teaching about that concept: "Excess leads to rejection."

We are all here to help each other reach that state of enlightenment. We know it brings balance and harmony into our own lives, and all that we come in contact with. The major drawback and problem with this concept of sacrifice is that the person is always thinking about others first. Doing for others what they should be doing for themselves is not a healthy pattern of behavior for either person. The person who is caught up in the pattern of sacrifice will often find they are also in the pattern of depletion. In this case, the depletion is in their health. Sometimes their money too. There is also the fact that in many cases, they neglect themselves. Making matters worse, no one is "feeding" them what they need. This, in turn, can lead to resentment. "I do for everyone, and no one does for me!" This resentment can lead to anger when they are not nourished or cared for in return. Anger and resentment, paired with frustration and guilt, are the emotional causes of cancer.

Seeing

The goal here is to know what kinds of scenes stimulate your need to get involved. There are some situations that resonate more with you than others. When these are seen, you feel the need to help in some way. You may even feel that you should do the project for the individual.

A different type of situation is this example: You get a call at some point in the evening, could be during dinner, while watching TV, reading, playing with the kids, or after you go to bed. The person on the other end of the line is a friend who, in truth, you are not really that close with. They "need a favor." They want you to pick them up and give them a ride home. They have family in the immediate area, but they called you. There are many reasons they did. Maybe the family members won't help because they know something you don't. Maybe the person is on the outs with the family. They have called you because they knew you are an easy mark. They know you will always avail yourself.

Listening

Much like seeing, you must become aware of those things said and implied that trigger your need to be involved—to the point of giving, giving, and giving more, but not getting anything in return. Of course, there are two things that happen here. The first is the religious aspect whispering, "It's your duty and obligation to help." This is true. We all have a responsibility to help our brothers and sisters. After all, we are all the children of God. However, this obligatory feeling can go too far in giving. This can trigger the second aspect: the need, want, or desire to be recognized for giving and wanting something in return. When this occurs, resentment and anger make evolve.

Thinking

Seeing and hearing the triggers that set this pattern in motion, it becomes clear that not responding is essential. You need to keep in mind that everything that happens to a person, including you, is set in motion by their/your mind. The actions and transactions occurring are a pattern of behavior at work. All patterns are designed to fulfill the expectation at the end of the cyclic flow of that pattern. The expectation that is being fulfilled validates the concept as being true, even when it is a misconception. Even when it works against you, like the pattern of sacrifice.

Program

I am not receptive to sacrifice. I am not making myself available to abuse. I am not allowing others to take advantage of me.

How does this pattern play out in the various Selves?
Emotional Self

Are you willing to give of Self?

Do you expect nothing in return?

Physical Self

Do you do for others to the point of depletion?

Material Self

Do you give financial aid to your detriment?

Social Self

Do you do everything for others and leave no time for Self?

Spiritual Self

Do you give and do for the church and people without taking care of Self?

SAVIOR

This particular pattern is shared by most parents, even those who laid the foundation for rejection in their children. These parents are the "knight on the white horse" coming to the rescue of their children. Of course, not every parent feels or acts this way. On some levels, this is the very opposite of "tough love." With tough love, the parent(s) just give up trying to help their child. I think that real tough love is sticking with the child and doing what you can without overly sacrificing yourself or being taken advantage of to help them through their crisis, no matter what!

There are many patterns that can come into play with this pattern. The thing to keep in mind is that you cannot save anyone but yourself. In this pattern, you must become, as Jesus taught in the Gospel According to Thomas 42, "a passerby." Learn to be an observer and walk on, especially of you feel it could threaten your emotional or physical health. It is not always necessary or appropriate to get involved with another person's pattern. The desire to help, rescue, and play the savior role serves one's ego, and rarely does it serve the person being "rescued." Save the "lifeguarding" for life-threatening situations! It's hard to do but creates proper boundaries and helps others learn to problem-solve for themselves.

In every situation that you become emotionally involved in, you lose a clear perspective. Your vision and feelings are influenced and shaded by your concepts. A familiar statement relating to this is "looking at things through rose-colored glasses. The Universal Teaching on having particular perceptions of people is found in Luke 6:41: "And why beholdest thou the mote that is in thy brother's eye, but perceivest not the beam that is in thine own eye?"

Seeing

This pattern is very easy to see in others but hard to see in the Self. When a parent engages in this pattern, they see it as being helpful. "It's my duty!" can also be heard. This statement is from the pattern of obligation, maybe sacrifice as well. Learn to see when you are participating or feel the need to intervene and resolve the situation. Keep in mind the person you want to save has created the situation for their own personal/ego/patternistic reasons. Buddha said, "No one saves us but ourselves. No one can and no one may. We ourselves must walk the path." Jesus had this to say about saving oneself: "If you bring forth what is within you, what you bring forth will save you. If you do not bring forth what is within you, what you do not bring forth will destroy you." The Gospel According to Thomas #70.

Listening

Having ears to hear is a critical tool that will help you stay on the path within to the Kingdom. So it is prudent that when a person calls out for help, you access the situation. Are they really asking you to save them? Or are they asking you to do it for them? In the same respect, you must listen to yourself and see if you are extending a helping hand or a crippling hand. If you fix their problem, then you diminish their courage and confidence in their own ability to handle things in the future.

Thinking

As stated above, it is easy to see and hear when someone wants you to rescue them. It is harder to see it in oneself. In thinking, you must use the gift of recall and question yourself: "Have I asked to be rescued from a current situation? Do I call on God/Jesus/Buddha/Shiva or a Higher Power to save me from what is occurring?" Don't feel bad if you do! You have been conditioned to ask for help. Man wants you dependent on him. Man wants you to believe that only through him can you get to God or Jesus. This is not true. Jesus taught: "Neither shall they say, Lo here! or, Lo there! For, behold, the Kingdom of God is within you" (Luke 17:21). Recall Genesis 1:26: "And God said, Let us make man in our image, after our likeness; and let them have dominion over the fish of the sea, and over the fowl of the air, and over the cattle, and over all the earth, and over every creeping thing that creepeth upon the earth."

Program

I am powerful. I am a part of the God Force and am thus endowed with personal power.

I am never placed in a situation that I cannot master. I draw on my past successes to master this current situation.

How does this pattern play out in the various Selves?
Emotional Self
Where does your doubt and lack of confidence come from that makes you feel you need outside help, or rescuing?
What do you say or do that causes others to be dependent upon you? Why do you feel good when you have rescued someone? Do you ever initiate problems for others so you can play the "lifeguard" and then jump in to rescue them?
Physical Self
What types of things are you dependent on to get through life?
If you like to play the hero and rescue others, how have you physically intervened in a person's life that was appropriate? How did you intervene in a way that was not appropriate?
Material Self
In what ways do you set up situations where you need rescuing?
In what ways do you let others know (especially children) that you will rescue them?
Social Self
What image have you created for yourself so that others look to you for help, for rescuing?
Spiritual Self
Do you constantly ask/pray for help?
Do you ask for salvation?

SELF-DESTRUCTION
Needless to say, this is a very devastating pattern. It can lead to great harm—including death. Some paths that lead down this slippery slope are alcohol, drugs, and wanton behavior. There are many reasons for the self-destruction pattern to manifest. Feelings of being unloved, unworthy, and the need for rejection are just a few main causes. Death is the ultimate form of rejection.

Seeing

The first step here is seeing and acknowledging that you are in that mode and on that path. This is hard to do. It's hard to accept that you are damaging yourself, your relationships, and your future. In fact, the hardest thing to do is to be honest with one's self. In applying seeing in this pattern, you need to become aware of two fundamental signs. The first is you are about to start down that path. Become aware of those actions you take, or were taken against you. That gives you the justification that you need to punish yourself or beat yourself up over something. The second is the awareness of gathering implements of destruction. These could be as simple as making sure you are never out of alcohol, cigarettes, your drugs of choice, and the items that facilitate the main sources of your self-destruction efforts.

Listening

Learning to hear the subtle signs that stimulate the pattern is essential. There are things that you say to yourself that will set you on the path. Here are a few examples: "It was a very hard day. I need a drink to relax." "I am feeling really down. I need a hit to feel better." "I really should not have done that. I feel guilty. I need to punish myself." There are things people say and do to you that will also start the ball rolling. When you hear or see something that triggers you, make a note of it. This begins your awareness and is worthy of another dictionary entry. Because the concepts and patterns are so entrenched, there will be many instances that will justify the employment of the pattern.

Thinking

In this aspect there is the gathering of the signs and actions that you take that stimulate the pattern into action. You must question the whys and wherefores of where the pattern is coming from. Which of your many concepts of Self is the foundation of this pattern? There are two reasons you have these concepts. The first is you brought some of it with you. By that, I mean it is a concept you are working on to remove from your soul/spirit as you continue your journey toward reunification with the God Force. In doing so, you also learned this concept from your mother or father. That will depend upon your gender. In this situation, I assume you are the opposite of your gender's roles, actions, and behaviors. This also reveals that you are probably using rejection as a form of acceptance. If the assessment is correct, that will also help you to begin to identify when and where you seek rejection. This is a whole other matter that requires examination and understanding.

Program

I am a part of the God Force. I am worthy. I am deserving of having good things in my life. I am a good person. I am exercising awareness and self-control over the pattern.

How does this pattern play out in the various Selves?

Emotional Self

How do you work against yourself?

What do you say or do that causes others to depart from your life?

Physical Self

What types of dangerous things do you do?

Do you seek to involve others?

Material Self

In what ways do you undermine your efforts at having a good life?

Social Self

What have you created that makes others not include you?

Spiritual Self

Have you turned away from God?

Have you turned away from Self?

SELFISHNESS

The pattern of selfishness is "all about me!" In this person's mind, they are the most important individual in any situation. They come first in every interaction. They will also indulge themselves in whatever they want. No expense is denied them!

Seeing

Seek to become aware of how and when you indulge yourself and act selfish. It could be as simple and as subtle as giving yourself a larger portion of food, snacks, or drinks. Maybe you took the last piece of desert, even though someone else in the household didn't get a single slice. Examine how you diminish your affections, resources, time, and attention to others. See how whatever is going to take place is usually done on your schedule, your clock, and at your demand. These are all signs of being self-centered. Another term often heard is egotistical.

Listening

The small voice in your head will speak to you on two levels: do it, or don't do it. In the do it conversation sits all the justification for taking the largest share, having your way, being sure you are not denied the lager piece. The don't do it voice is the one of reason and thoughtfulness. Sometimes it reaches the surface before your ego shuts it down. Listen to the comments others may say in a joking fashion. They may outright call you selfish. You may laugh it off; nonetheless, they told you what they thought. Learn to listen and act accordingly, sharing and giving freely to others in order to become the new caring, thoughtful you.

Thinking

In this application you need to understand why you have a desire or need to be selfish. Do you think that in the past you were denied something, so now you make sure you get your share? Again, you must ask yourself, "Who do I take after?" This will help you let go of this pattern. After all, it works against you becoming a better person. Another aspect of thinking is seeking to discover the concept that uses this pattern as a means of maintaining access to "the doorway home."

Program

I am sharing more and more. I am giving freely of my abundance. I am listening more. I am allowing others to be the center of attention. I am becoming more loving.

How does this pattern play out in the various Selves?

Emotional Self

Are you a taker instead of a giver, or are you one who shares with others?

Physical Self

Do you try to get all that is available to you, such as food, money, and attention?

Material Self

Do you try to get it all?

Does money drive you? What do you think money will do for you?

Social Self

Do you not enjoy sharing the limelight?

Do you make yourself the center of conversation?

Spiritual Self

Do you think it's all about you?

Do you think God only looks out for you?

SELF-PITY

This pattern can be used as a means of garnering attention. It can appear by getting others to come to your rescue. It is, on some levels, a cry for help. "Woe is me! Please help."

Seeing

Here, it is beneficial to see the things you set in motion to create a situation where self-pity will manifest. An example might be going to an ATM machine, inserting your card, the computer glitching out, signaling that you have no money. To top it off, the machine does not return your card. Another more common example would be knowing that a friend is throwing a party, but you are not invited. Keep in mind that you are the creator of everything that happens to you. Every action and reaction you are experiencing is the result of your concepts and the patterns of behavior you demonstrate.

Listening

This aspect provides you opportunities to learn when the self-pity energy is starting to evolve from the subconscious. You may get into a conversation with yourself about how bad things are in your life. Someone offended you, or you were neglected by your best friend. These are a few examples of signs your mind gives, alerting you that something else has triggered the need for self-pity. The "something elses" are the things you must become attuned to stop this pattern from derailing you.

Thinking

A good place to begin is asking yourself, "How does indulging in self-pity work for me? What benefits do I derive? How does it serve me?" These answers and others that you will come upon will be great guidance in overcoming this detrimental pattern. Another aspect of thinking is seeking to discover the concept that uses this pattern as a means of maintaining access to "the doorway home."

Program

I am strong. I am handling whatever comes my way. I am aware of self-pity indulgences. I am eliminating self-pity from my life. I am a part of God.

How does this pattern play out in the various Selves?

Emotional Self

Do you do things, or set things in motion, to have people feel sorry for you?

Especially those very close to you?

What do you do to get that need satisfied?

Physical Self

Do you hurt yourself?

Do you complain constantly about an ailment that you have?

Do you overwork yourself when you work out, creating injuries?

Do you have a tendency to have accidents?

Material Self

Do you end up making bad investments or lose money easily?

Do you break things that have to be replaced?

Social Self

What things do you say to get your friends and family involved in your pity-party?

Spiritual Self

Do you feel abandoned because your prayers are not answered?

Do you feel you are not worthy of having your prayers answered?

SUCCESS & FAILURE

This pattern is employed by those with great potential; however, within their subconscious mind they believe that in being successful they will be rejected from the doorway back to the spiritual plane. To ensure their return, they will create situations that lead to denying themselves completion and success because that achievement is not in keeping with their mom's expectation of their persona. That is not to say that Mom is the problem. After all, the child chose that set of parents because it offered their soul an opportunity to understand and master an aspect of themselves in order to move forward. Keep in mind that everything comes back to the Self.

When a new opportunity is presented, the person in the success and failure pattern will move on it. However, as time goes by, they may include elements that will undermine future moves. These elements (be they people, procedures, or policies) may create a depletion, thus stopping forward movement. Of course, there will be a logical, rational, and justifiable reason not to continue.

Seeing

When something occurs that requires attention, there will be an attitude of "I will get to that." Because it is not dealt with when it should have been, the person sets themself up for trouble and possibly failure. Another sign is when something is presented that appears to be a good idea because of price, or perceived benefit, and is pursued without further investigation. This could lead to depletion (which is another pattern of behavior) of one's finances and resources, thus setting the stage for failure.

Lastly, an example that you are going into the pattern toward failure (incompletion), is seeing something that reminds you of something similar in the past that led to incompletion, procrastination, denial, or avoidance toward handling a situation. It could be a person, an email, a letter, a phone call, or even a smell. These are all signs your mind is drawing your attention to in an effort to make you aware. This becomes an opportunity to add to your personal dictionary. Your mind is always talking to you in your unique language via signs, icons, and symbols. All of these manifestations are designed to keep you on the narrow path that leads to the true life. Here is the Universal Teaching on this: "Narrow is the way, which leadeth unto life, and few there be that find it" (Matthew 7:14). Many followers of Christianity think that because they are Christian, they have found "the path." They have not, unless they have looked and journeyed within to the Kingdom of God. "Neither shall they say, Lo here! or, Lo there! For, behold, the Kingdom of God is within you" (Luke 17:21).

Listening

Listening is a twofold ally. It can work for you or against you. Your mind will talk to you as "the quiet voice in your head," coming from the Spiritual Self to provide an insight. It may tell you, "This is not a good thing to do. This is something to investigate. Do you really trust this person, opportunity, situation?" And you choose to ignore it. That is setting yourself up for failure. On the other hand, you may talk yourself into something because it fulfills your need to fail. Of course, this is the end result of motivation to fulfill the exception of Self as being a failure. Another form of listening is what people say to you. Some may say, "Great idea!" knowing that it can't be done by you, for one reason or another. You must learn to hear what people say and intuiting their intent. I know you have heard the expression, "Not everything (seen or heard) is what it appears to be." That is great advice. Take it to heart.

Thinking

This is where you set in motion the failure part of the pattern. You may think of something and believe it is the greatest thing since sliced bread. You embark upon that thought until halfway through, when you realize it can't be done for one reason or another. You have spent a lot of money, time, and energy on it. The time took you away from other endeavors that could a have been more productive. This is also where you come up with the reasons not to continue (after all, it just might take you to success). Your reasons will be sound, based on a logical, rational, and or justifiable assumption. Another aspect of thinking is seeking to discover the concept that uses this pattern as a means of maintaining access to "the doorway home."

Program

I am drawing on past successes. I am in control of my emotions. I am aware of distractions. I am a part of God and have what I need to succeed.

How does this pattern play out in the various Selves?
Emotional Self

What attributes do you possess that can lead to great happiness? Empathy? Compassion? Kindness? Openness?

Do you always "turn away" at the last minute? Do you turn away from a relationship?

Can you not keep a relationship going?

Do you reject an opportunity for growth?

Are you quick to reject others?

Do you create situations to be rejected?

Physical Self

What attributes do you possess that can lead to great health?

Do you have a good genetic background?

Are you athletic? Nicely toned?

Is it difficult to stay on a diet? Do you indulge in junk food?

Do you eat excessive amounts of sugar and carbohydrates?

The Universal Teaching for this is: "Excess leads to rejection." Also, read Buddha's directive: "To keep the body in good health is a duty . . . otherwise we shall not be able to keep our mind strong and clear."

Material Self

What attributes do you possess that can lead to great financial success?

Education? Skill? Creative expression?

Do you often not deal with situations? Issues?

Do you create situations to get yourself fired?

Do you create situations that make you want to quit?

Do you not complete tasks? Not finish tasks/projects in timely manner?

Do you have frequent delays in turning in your work?

Have you made bad investments? Do you gamble?

Do you have an addiction, such as a drug habit?

Social Self

What attributes do you possess that can lead to great successes? Great personality?

Are you intelligent? A conversationalist?

Do you create a habit that stimulates rejection from others?

Do you say inappropriate things or attack people verbally?

Do you stir the pot? Meaning, do you always say something to create an argument?

The Universal Teaching in line with success and failure is, "There is nothing from without a man, that entering into him can defile him; but the things which come out of him, [things said] those are they that defile the man" (Mark 7:15).

Spiritual Self

What attributes do you possess that can lead to great peace within?

Are you able to be alone?

Are you able to focus?

Do you struggle to go within to understand the Self?

"If you bring forth what is within you,
what you bring forth will save you.
If you do not bring forth what is within you,
what you do not bring forth will destroy you."
—The Gospel According to Thomas 70.

"Peace comes from within.
Do not seek it without."
—Buddha

WITHDRAWAL

This pattern is more obvious than others. Here, the person may feel inadequate, unattractive, have nothing to say or share, and feel safer being by themself than amongst others. One example may be that the person has been denigrated at home, thus undermining their confidence. Another is being bullied at school. Another could be the lack of social graces, such as not being able to dance. There are many reasons for these feelings and actions. It is necessary to gain control over them.

Seeing

With the withdrawal pattern, it is important to become aware of the signs and things that trigger the desire to be alone or withdraw form a conversation. It could be as simple as the way someone looks at you. It may make you feel inadequate or unattractive. You need to always understand what you are looking at and how it is affecting you. Seeing something that bothers you and not speaking up creates emotional turmoil within. That turmoil can lead to disease, especially if it is anger because anger is one emotional cause of cancer.

Listening

Like seeing, listening relates to hearing what someone says and those words may trigger feelings of inferiority; thus stimulating the need to withdraw from the conversation, event, or the relationship. Here, it is important to learn to identify those triggering words so that you become immune to them and the resultant action of withdrawing.

Thinking

It is imperative to understand where this motivation to withdraw comes from. Who are you emulating? Or is it a question of who "beat" you into doubt and uncertainty of your worth? Withdrawal is an aspect of doubt and fear manifesting differently. Another aspect of thinking is seeking to discover the concept that uses this pattern as a means of maintaining access to "the doorway home."

Program

I am gaining more courage every day. I am becoming more confident in myself. I am speaking up more. I am getting more involved in life.

How does this pattern play out in the various Selves?
Emotional Self

What causes you to pull away from people?
What causes you to avoid entanglements?

Physical Self

Do you withdraw from sports or other activities?

What are the thoughts behind this attitude of physical withdrawal?

Material Self

Do you feel unworthy to have things?

Do you feel undeserving? Do you feel incapable?

Does your withdrawing keep you in poverty-mode?

Social Self

Do you have feelings of inferiority? Where do they come from?

Who makes you feel inferior?

Are you reclusive?

Spiritual Self

Do you not want to participate in family beliefs? Are you an unbeliever?

What turns you off? Do you like feel you don't have what it takes?

Discipline of Discipline

The origin of the word "discipline" is from the Latin *disciplina*, which means "instruction or knowledge." That is the true purpose of discipline, to create a particular way of thinking. This is also why the twelve apostles are considered to be the disciples of Jesus, because it is a particular way of thinking and acting. Thinking comes before acting because all outward actions are based on internal thought processes. Thoughts are created in the subconscious mind for the purpose of validating subconscious concepts we maintain. The thought then sets in motion the thinking process.

There are multiple definitions of the word discipline. In addition to a way of gathering knowledge, another interpretation indicates the practice of training people to obey rules. To that end, I think all of us have been disciplined as children so we would follow and obey the rules and regulations. When we didn't there was a punishment.

Discipline can also represent a particular code of behavior. This can manifest as social convention all the way to military correctness. The fourth is a way of thinking, a new discipline (sociology or astrology). These four applications are forms of disciplines. In examining the definitions of the word discipline, the last one was a "new discipline." That's what I would like to present to you in this book: A new discipline. A new way of thinking. A new way of experiencing life.

Another definition is with respect to creating a habit, a habitual way of doing something. In this case, we are going to talk about twelve specific disciplines. As you incorporate the disciplines into your life and make them a habit, you will manifest them as a manner of *being*, which will further your growth and allow you to accomplish the things you truly desire. It will also allow you to control and eliminate the negative occurrences in your personal history.

I mentioned earlier that another form of discipline is punishment. Interestingly, people punish themselves. When you do something you shouldn't have and then feel guilty about it, you end up creating a situation that will literally bring to light whatever transacted. This is done in order for you to bring the authorities upon you. The authorities could be Mom, Dad, your wife, or the law. You may also create a disunity or disharmony and ultimately end up with a punishment. We are not going to concentrate on "setups," but I did want to bring it up so you can understand why certain things happen to you. It is you creating the situation. It is no one else's fault.

Here is a Universal Teaching found in Mathew 7:7 that relates to this: "For everyone that asketh receiveth." People do not realize that everything they ask for at a subconscious level they will receive. It is through this transaction that each of us are co-creating our personal reality. In the first definition of discipline, we defined it as the practice of doing something repeatedly in a particular way, a habit. The beauty of developing a habit is that it becomes a discipline. You create a program in your mind, much like a bio-computer, and it runs automatically. When you create particular disciplines, they will also run automatically.

The benefit of a discipline is that it will help you achieve your goals. In terms of goals, I would have you set four different goals, since there are four aspects of the Self. The Spiritual Self is the one through which all communication begins from the Creator that dwells within.

Neither shall they say, Lo here! Or, lo there!
for, behold, the kingdom of God is within you.
—Luke 17:21

The directives that come from your Spiritual Self lead you toward balance and harmony in the most spiritual of ways. The problem arises when you seek to manifest that directive. It must first pass through your Emotional Self. Therein lies the corruption. The Emotional Self has its own agenda. All of its actions are designed to gain acceptance from Mother because she is the way into the material plane. The material plane is the third dimension where we live. On the flip side, there is the spiritual plane.

The spiritual plane is where we come from, where we dwell prior to entering into the material plane. The purpose of the material plane is to cleanse the soul of all manmade concepts so that one can evolve out of the material plane into the next level of spiritual evolution. Jesus is the example in mastering death. So we know death can be mastered. It is all a matter of understanding. At a deep, subconscious level everyone believes that their mother is the only way back to the spiritual plane; therefore acceptance is essential.

Creating a Discipline

To create a discipline is very simple. It depends upon what you want to accomplish. For instance, suppose you want to paint, write, or sculpt, but you have a full-time job that is not what you really want to do. We all have to earn a living and keep a roof over our heads and feed our families. However, one of the most important things we should strive to do is to develop and grow our personal expression.

If you want to be a writer, I'll offer my daily discipline: In the morning while I am having my tea, I play Solitaire on my computer. This is part of my discipline because I believe that the mind needs to be exercised on a daily basis, above and beyond the work that I do. There should be exercises for both body and mind for the simple reason that the mind is like a muscle.

The muscular tone of the body can become flaccid and weak if you are not using it. The mind is in the same category. You need to exercise it. Use it or lose it. Exercise is so wonderful on many different levels. When you physically exercise, you oxygenate your body, which accomplishes two things. First, you are feeding your mind, 25 percent of all the oxygen you bring into your body is relegated to your brain. Now you are feeding your brain the key nutrient it requires for optimal functionality and cognition.

Second, when you oxygenate your blood, you oxygenate your body. Cancer and other types of anaerobic diseases are not able to establish themselves in an oxygen-rich environment. Another benefit, not so much oxygen driven, is that exercising burns fat and cholesterol, thus opening your arteries and allowing better circulation.

After my morning tea, I go to the gym and work out. Then I'm off to work. I get in around ten o'clock and work until four or five o'clock, depending on my work load. After that, I head back home were its news time, then dinner. Next, I watch *Wheel of Fortune* and *Jeopardy*, again from a mind-stimulating point of view. At 7:00 I go into my office for my scheduled writing time. At 9:00 I shut down, relax for an hour, watch some television, then go to bed at ten o'clock. That is my disciplined routine on a daily basis. I suggest that you examine your reality and see where you can instill habits and disciplines that will allow you to grow your expression, whatever it may be. It doesn't matter what it is, as long as you make an effort to grow something within yourself other than a disease or condition.

The bottom line with creating a discipline is to first make up your mind to do it. Know that there will be multiple distractions to try to keep you from creating a discipline. Why? The answer is simple: your Emotional Self does not believe that you can grow beyond where you are. To validate that your Emotional Self will set up everything it can to keep you where you are, thus proving that you cannot move forward. Here is where your personal history is at work. This is not true. You can become what you want to be. You just have to work at it.

I've previously written about friends coming and going in your life. Some are there for the long haul and some for a short period of time. As I stated, they are just symbolic of a cycle you are going through at the time. So they become a sign to help you understand a pattern at work, a pattern that is part of your personal history.

From a different point of view, you could consider your Emotional Self as a friend, but one of negative influence to your Spiritual Self, which is your friend-friend, the one who wants you to succeed and move forward, to grow and evolve. But your Emotional-Self friend wants to hold you back because it is comfortable with the relationship where it is. Sometimes you have to end a relationship. The way that you do it when it comes to the Emotional Self is through understanding what the relationship is built on, which are your subconscious concepts. Therefore they need to be understood and controlled so they have no impact in your life.

A major distraction is the concept that discipline means restriction or confinement. With that belief, the person will resist the authority to impose a discipline, even on themselves. This concept is part of the rejection for acceptance patterns. In truth, it works against the person because it is only through discipline that you can master anything, especially your Self. Keep in mind that God never places you in a situation that you cannot handle or master, no matter the situation, disease, condition, relationship, etc.

"There hath no temptation taken you but such as is common to man:
but God is faithful, who will not suffer you to be tempted
above that ye are able; but will with the temptation also
make a way to escape, that ye may be able to bear it."
—1 Corinthians 10:13

Whatever situation you encounter, you can handle it, and when you understand it, you can begin to control it. Emotional control will lead you to physical mastery. Remember, a discipline or habit can be a tool for helping you accomplish whatever you want to accomplish in this life.

The Discipline of Thought

What are thoughts? Where do they come from? To better understand the concept as generally accepted, here is a definition of *thought* from Wikipedia: "Thought can refer to the ideas or arrangements of ideas that result from thinking, the act of producing thoughts, or the process of producing thoughts." Although thought is a fundamental human activity familiar to everyone, there is no generally accepted agreement as to what thought is or how it is created. Thoughts are the result or product of either spontaneous or willed acts of thinking.

Because thought underlies many human actions and interactions, understanding its physical and metaphysical origins, processes, and effects has been a longstanding goal of many academic disciplines, including psychology, neuroscience, philosophy, artificial intelligence, biology, sociology, and cognitive science.

Note that when you are reading signs, omens, and symbols, the moment you "get it" is when you generate/create a thought. This thought springs from a particular concept in your subconscious mind. A concept has been stimulated and has become active. Upon that awareness of a sign/symbol, the mind goes into thinking to see how to carry out that subconscious thought, the end result, the need, want, desire. Now a pattern of behavior has just been set in motion. Actions follow thought, with thinking as the facilitator.

To continue the definition of *thought*: "Thinking allows humans to make sense of, interpret, represent or model the world they experience, and to make predictions about that world. It is therefore helpful to an organism with needs, objectives, and desires as it makes plans or otherwise attempts to accomplish those goals."

Thinking is the process of thoughts forming a plan of action for achieving its goal. Thinking is an interesting gift, even though we never think of it as such. It goes without saying that all of us *think*. What is meant here in these writings is to take it deeper. We look at many things and maybe we give them a quick thought, or not, and we move on because everything seems fine.

However, there are times when you hear or see a sign and you must stop immediately and start thinking what it is your mind is saying to you. You need to discern what's taking place. What are the present energies stimulating concepts within your subconscious mind? What patterns of behavior are about to be set in motion? You need to see what energies are aligned and working against you. They will come from internal and then external forces. The Discipline of Observation must be employed first to read the sign/symbol. Then think. Take your time to think and read the symbol from as many angles as you can. Relate everything back to yourself. The best understanding of a symbol is the one you relate to on a personal, emotional level.

Some good "thinking" questions might be: *What is going on? What am I involved in? Where am I going? What is upcoming? What do I have to deal with?* These questions will stimulate certain conversations within, as well they should. By taking an assessment of everything that is going on and everything you are dealing with, you now have an understanding of where you are in the unfolding of particular patterns.

Knowing where you are may help you through the process of taking thinking to the next level to understand why you are there. Once that is understood, then you can apply the understanding to it, knowing that it is going to take change on your part to get to where you want to go.

THE 4 Ps

The next thing to start thinking about is a plan of action. There are ways to plan that will ensure success. The 4 Ps will offer the greatest chance of success: Plan, Prepare, Project and Provide.

:**PLAN** For whatever it is that you are seeking to accomplish, you need to have a plan of action. Think through every aspect and the steps that need to be taken, then write down your plan.

:**PREPARE** As Confucius said, "Success is dependent upon preparation; no matter the project, preparation is the key." Now that you have an idea of what you need to implement the Plan, ask yourself, "Does it require licensing? Does it require special training? Does it require special tools?" Think of every step along the way and what is required. Preparations will give you the stability to move up to the next step.

:**PROJECT** Project ahead as far as you can see, and make notes of everything that you know you will have to deal with. You may see some things that require greater preparation, and that is why projecting is vital. The next area to project into is the Self. What within you would keep you from manifesting your goal? Are there particular concepts telling you that you are not entitled, that you lack authority or are not worthy, and that you do not deserve it? Do you have a tendency to procrastinate? Be aware of what is within, because that may work against you in completing your goal.

Visualize your goal, and if it is a concept, write it out. Even a concept has some aspects of manifestation that you would like to attain. Visualize that and understand it. Fortify your mind with such intent so that it becomes virtually invulnerable.

PROVIDE: Providing addresses the Self. It is easy enough to gather materials to understand the requirements and whatever it is that you need. The hard part is knowing your role and how it is that you act and react in certain projects. Providing is done on multiple levels. First, go over your checklist and make sure every contingency of the planning stage has been addressed. Do you have everything? Have you provided for everything that is required by city, county, state, federal government? Also, examine those things you need to understand and be aware of based on your concepts and patterns.

Reexamine your projections, both outward and inward. Inward is the more important, because what you have to provide is the understandings where uncertainty, doubt, and fear operate. You can curtail their influence by being aware of how they may try to manifest in whatever the project is so that you look at all angles and all levels. Provide for all of that, and you are in a position of strength to move forward.

The Path Forward

Moving forward requires thinking. It can also incorporate or lead to the further development of the spiritual gift of Clairvoyance. The reason being the more you think, the deeper you get into the energy of something, the more likely you are to flow with it. From that vantage point, you have a glimpse of its essence and, possibly, what the future may hold. This could also manifest as the spiritual gift of Prophecy.

Another gift associated with thinking, from one point of view, is Perseverance. Perseverance exists on different levels. You can persevere because you have to, and that might lead to resentment. Or you can persevere out of determination going through obstacles in order to achieve your goal.

As a gift, perseverance teaches stamina and helps one to build strength. If you have to persevere through a situation, you are constantly thinking about the easiest, fastest way to get it done that meets your needs. Your needs are either going to be seeking approval or rejection, and your mind will work to set up either event in order to validate the end need.

Perseverance will provide strength that will help you to have the stamina and the courage necessary to persevere through whatever is presented to you. Remember, you co-created the event, situation, or illness. Therefore you are the solution and cure. All you need do is understand what is going on and then make the necessary adjustments on every level to create the reality you want.

A fifth P was suggested to me by a student and practitioner of this work: Patience. This is a characteristic you must have, and if you feel you lack patience, then make it a priority to develop and practice this attribute.

The Discipline of Emotions

What are the emotions? How do they work? Why do we have them? These are questions that need to be understood. With that in mind, here is what a dictionary gave as the definition of emotions: "A natural, instinctive state of mind deriving from one's circumstances, mood, or relationships with others; instinctive or intuitive feeling as distinguished from reasoning or knowledge."

In the first definition we see that emotions are stimulated by others. This is where we will need to understand how others affect us. Depending on what your need may be emotionally, that would be your area of vulnerability. The goal is to know the things that trigger you through reading signs, symbols, and listening to what people say. Know what it is that triggers your emotional responses in both a positive and negative way. The more you can understand that, the more you can have a great relationship while at the same time maintaining emotional control.

In the second definition we see more of an ethereal understanding. In many ways we would relate this definition to "chemistry." It is something we immediately experience and know that we are experiencing it. Examples would be walking into a room and "reading the energy." Meeting someone for the first time and immediately hitting it off as if you were old friends is another example.

The first definition is where the effects may not surface immediately but are working in your subconscious mind, setting in motion patterns of behavior appropriate for the concept stimulated. Once the pattern is set in motion, it will seek to prove whatever concept has been triggered as being true.

Many of the concepts people have in their subconscious mind are man-made ideals, standards, and values that are not necessarily in keeping with the truth of the Universal Teachings, the laws of God. Learning to control emotions is a difficult task for several reasons. On one level, it is your emotions that attach you, along with your senses, to the material plane. To see this in action visualize yourself standing still with a gazillion threads of energy emanating from you in all directions. Also see everyone else doing the same thing, emanating threads like lines of power. It is through your emotional threads you are connected to everyone, and to material reality.

When the emotions get out of control, they can lead to chaos. You hear so many stories in the news where perhaps a couple is arguing and someone will intervene to stop the argument and ends up dead. Things like that happen for many different reasons, including karma.

Emotions run the gamut from love to hatred—and every emotion in between. Going back to our thread example, I want you to visualize the same gazillion threads coming out of you in all directions. When you are angry or experiencing the base emotion of hatred, it looks like billions of those lines converging in one area toward one object or situation. Each convergence would be different. In this case it is hatred, so the threads are black and aggressive. If you are experiencing love, then I want you to visualize millions of light-infused threads radiating outward from your body in all directions. This is what is happening energetically, so tuning into this experience allows you to recognize the power of your emotions affecting the space and people around you.

The emotions can lead to entanglements—some good and some bad; some productive and some harmful. An entanglement is also known as a *quantum entanglement*, which has no distance barrier. It's the phenomena of two separate particles (from different sources) affecting the other. This is the unavoidable consequence of living in an entangled and interconnected physical and spiritual reality. One has to be mindful of one's emotional outreach as well as one's emotional receptivity.

The Discipline of Manifestation

You are already manifesting your reality. You are co-creating your reality with God who dwells within. What you are experiencing is a result of what your subconscious concepts are shaping in your life at this moment. There is a Universal Teaching that relates to this statement.

> "Jesus said: Know what is in thy sight and
> what is hidden from thee will be revealed to thee.
> For there is nothing hidden which will not be made manifest."
> —*The Gospel According to Thomas* 5

All of us have certain concepts in our subconscious mind that tell us who it is we think we should be and how we should act. Depending upon your age, most of us have that so deeply ingrained that it is an automatic position one adheres to in life. That does not necessarily mean that it is a good thing, because one must evolve.

You would think that we are talking about manifesting the reality you want. And we are. However, it also refers to your own personal spiritual growth, because the more you understand yourself, the more you allow the Spiritual Self to manifest. As faith in Self grows, so does your ability to master the material plane.

There are many books written on how to manifest whatever you want. A quick approach to manifesting anything is using deep meditation to program your mind with "I am" statements, such as "I am becoming wealthy" or "I am becoming rich" or whatever it is you want to accomplish, including health. If you precede whatever your desire with the expression "I AM," you are telling God within you to work for you in accomplishing what you want. The "I AM" is one of the many names of God. It was first stated when Moses was in front of the burning bush and asked God, "Who should I say sent me?" God answered, "I AM that I AM" (Exodus 3:14).

Another technique for manifesting what you want is through visualization. In this approach, you see what you want in your mind's eye—your imagination. At the same time you are pouring energy into the visualization, do your programming. In this way, you are reenforcing what you want. You can certainly use this technique for healing, except in your mind's eye I invite you to see the part you are seeking to heal in perfect health so that your brain knows what to do. Make sure you are giving it the "food" it needs to do whatever it is you want it to do. Food can be many things, such as self-encouragement, exercise, and a great diet so you have the stamina and endurance to carry you through your endeavor. Another resource to consider are quality nutritional supplements as a way of fortifying the body.

You must be strong on all levels and in as many areas as is possible to accomplish your goals. You must also understand yourself to keep what you create. Perhaps you have heard stories of people who win the lottery, and three years later they are flat broke or suffered a tragedy and lost everything.

You hear of people who have attended positive thinking seminars and after a couple of cycles, everything seems to be working as it should. Then their momentum and results disappear. Part of the answer is karma. That is why some have it easy, or so it appears. However, what appears to be easy may also be very difficult to break away from. Another reason for the decline in results is that the person becomes immersed in the culture, traditions, and attachment to the material plane to such a degree that the Spiritual Self does not fully grow and develop and does not express all of the gifts that it has.

The Discipline of Cycles

Everything in the universe flows in cycles. A quick example is our planet circling the sun. This gives us four seasons. What is interesting is that we have four Selves, as mentioned earlier: The Spiritual Self is where everything begins. The Emotional Self is where things are set in motion to manifest our desired reality. The Physical Self (Material Self) relates to the body and health. The material aspect is the physical reality, which includes lifestyle and possessions. This aspect of Self is a reflection of your subconscious concepts and beliefs in action.

The Social Self is how people interact with each other. Each of these Selves have particular concepts that relate to them. When any one of them is triggered or stimulated, the manifestation will be created through patterns of behavior that will lead to a specific result. This will validate the concept as true.

There are four cycles that you flow through in your patterns of behavior. They are the same as your four Selves. Because of the cycles, your personal history constantly repeats itself. When you begin to glimpse a pattern or see history repeating, it may benefit you to start a journal about your personal history. Think about things that happened to you, then see if you can remember the age you were, who you were with, and what was taking place at the time.

A simple example might be about friendships and relationships. See what they tell you. You may find that there are two types of friends. Those you have known for decades and those who come and go. Those that come and go happen during a particular cycle in your life that you were going through emotionally. Those people became symbols to you.

An example of this is when you bump into someone in the supermarket, or you get a postcard, letter, email, or phone call from someone you haven't spoken to in years. All of those happenings are your mind's way of using signs to tell you what you are going through at that very moment in time. Knowing what is taking place in the now gives you the opportunity to alter the future. You can make it what you want through understanding, application, and perseverance.

Relationships are a bit different in the sense that there is generally a deeper emotional connection. But even there, look at the relationships you have had, the nature of the relationships, and how long they have lasted. By understanding and recognizing the cyclic nature of them, the understanding will give you an indication of the kind of emotional things you go through on a cyclical basis. Once you begin to identify your cycles, they will help you pinpoint the pattern of behavior since the cycle is the vehicle. However, the pattern of behavior is the driver. It is always good to be mindful of cycles to understand where you are so that instead of your cycles running horizontally, like wheels on the ground, you can control the flow and direct it upward into a spiral.

By exercising control through reading signs and symbols, you are more on a cyclic spiral heading upward into higher levels of awareness and consciousness, manifesting more of your Spiritual Self. If you look at the construction of a spiral going up, you see it gets smaller. It is the same as a whirlpool upside down where it sucks everything into it. In this case, what it is doing is drawing your Spiritual Self up higher and higher, closer to unification with the Creative Continuum called God.

All personal cycles flow in the same sequence that the Self evolve. An example of this is how a baby develops into a child. Their cycles are spiritual, emotional, physical, and social. In the beginning, when the baby first comes into the material plane, it is truly more spiritual than emotional.

If you have ever been around children when they are being breast-fed or bottle-fed, you can see them staring up and following something in the room, an energy that we no longer see. But because the baby is new to this dimension, he or she still has the ability to see energies and ethereal bodies.

There is a Universal Teaching that hints to this awareness. It is found in the *The Gospel According to Thomas* 4:

> "Jesus said: "The man old in days will not hesitate to
> ask a little child of seven days about the place of Life,
> and he will live.
> For many who are first shall become last
> and they shall become a single one.""

Now we see the baby begins to make an effort to communicate within the first three months. The next three months involve more communication, and the baby is emoting more than before. The next three months the baby is beginning to become mobile and gaining control over its faculties. During months nine through twelve, the child is now interacting with parents and others, better able to communicate so that there is an understanding and a back-and-forth. Those are the four cycles in every cycle you go through; spiritual, emotional, physical (material), and social/intellectual.

The spiritual gift associated with cycles is Prophesy, because once you can begin to see your patterns at work within your cycles and understand them, it will help you grow your awareness and consciousness to be able to see larger cycles, societal cycles. You may even be able to see how particular national societies around the world are being patternistic in their behaviors. There is a Universal Teaching in Ecclesiastes 3:15:

"That which hath been is now;
and that which is to be hath already been;
and God requireth that which is past."

This Universal Teaching demonstrates that humankind is in an ongoing, repeating reality. This will continue on a personal level until one can understand the nature of it and thus gain control over it and have the cycles manifest differently.

In understanding what is going on, one can speculate and postulate what is potentially going to happen. The certainty, from a different point of view, is that if enough people believe it, then they all collectively bring it to be. That is not to say that the person professing something is not correct. There statement is more of a validation.

The Discipline of Observation

What is the purpose of observation? We all have eyes that see, except for those who are blind from birth or from an accident or disease. We have the ability to observe so we can see how to move forward without hurting ourselves on many levels and, on some levels, to keep others from hurting themselves. That is its basic purpose, to keep you on that narrow path that leads to life.

> "Enter ye in at the strait gate, for wide is the gate,
> and broad is the way,
> that leadeth to destruction,
> and many there be which go in thereat.
> Because strait is the gate,
> and narrow is the way,
> which leadeth unto life,
> and few there be that find it."
> —Matthew 7:13–14

The definition of observation is a process of observing something or someone in order to gain information. This information is designed to provide you guidance. The purpose being to harmonize the Self with the Creative Continuum called God. This is the Spiritual Energetic Flow that permeates everything.

The benefits of observation are simple. By seeing what is taking place, such as an action that someone is doing or a reaction you are having, observing allows you the opportunity to change your reaction to what is taking place through the process of questioning. This occurs as you change the energy within, which ultimately changes the energy without. This means, from a different point of view, that you will be able to accomplish what it is that you want to accomplish without the Emotional Self interfering and getting in the way. There are four different types of observations:

The Casual Eye

The casual perspective is how most people live their lives. Most see without really paying attention to the intent or message they are observing. On one level you are seeing everyday life and its occurrences. At the same time, your mind is using available items, situations, and events to "talk" to you. Woven into your daily life are occurrences where you may stub your toe, drop a glass, lose your keys or wallet, or get a ticket—and more subtle things. These signs and symbols are given to help you determine which pattern is at work and where in the cycle of its fulfillment you are. In the domain of observation is where you create your personal symbolic language. It begins with you tying together an emotional experience with a solid object. This process creates your unique symbolic language. These will be the signs you will use for guidance as life moves on.

You will create a Personal Emotional Association (PEA) with a symbol. It will be these signs and symbols that will provide the greatest guidance. Your mind is already using symbols to talk to you; however, you are not seeing or hearing them because you were not taught about signs, omens, or symbols as a form of communication. Nor do you know how to use them; therefore the guidance they provide often goes unheeded.

The universal interpretations that are offered through my book *The Dream Symbology Dictionary*, available at www.innerhealthbooks.com, will get you started. Once you have a basic understanding of the language is when you will add this information to your personal dictionary. You will know when your mind is talking to you. It is when you pay attention to something for more than half a second. If it catches your eye, that is your mind telling you something.

Your mind is talking to you every single day, if not every hour or minute. It depends on what you are involved in, what is going on, which particular pattern of behavior is in action, and which pattern has just been stimulated based on what you have observed. This is where the language of symbols and signs comes into play.

On the surface it all looks normal. However, with the Discipline of Observation you learn to see the energy and thought behind what is taking place. This is the living language of your mind. This is how your mind communicates with you.

A symbol can be anything from a sensation (Discipline of Touch), a vision (Discipline of Observation), or a smell (Discipline of Sensing). Symbols are associated with an emotional feeling that has been stimulated by what you have observed or experienced. You can observe something and have the smell of chocolate in the air come to mind. What you do when that occurs is the question: What do you associate with the smell of chocolate in the air with? It may be when your grandmother cooked chocolate chip cookies, you could smell it wafting through the house.

Now you think back and ask yourself: What did your grandmother making chocolate chip cookies represent to you at the time. It could be a sense of love, security, or simply a treat. Let's assume it was a treat. Perhaps what you just saw (a symbol) that triggered that particular memory is telling you that what you are seeking is a treat.

Then you question why is there a need for a treat. What is going on that you feel the need to reward yourself? Maybe the chocolate chip cookies were a comfort food. So what is taking place that you have this need for comfort? Observation helps you to identify where you are in a particular pattern of behavior and where you are in its cyclic flow. With this understanding, it gives you the opportunity to change the outcome. This helps you get closer to being the you that you want to be!

The Keen Eye

You may have heard the phrase "a keen eye." The word *keen* means "eagerness or enthusiasm." The keen eye is a has a unique and particular perspective. In fact, in the definition given, it implies "eagerness or enthusiasm," as in opportunities. You really do have to have a keen perspective, a different type of a perception when you are seeking an opportunity.

It is the same thing in everyday life. Every day you need to develop a keen eye to get past the casual look. The casual look only sees the surface. The clinical look, another type of observation, is similar to what a keen eye is; however, it is a little different in the sense that the keen eye is one that is more emotionally involved. The involvement is created because eagerness and enthusiasm are spiritual energies that ride on the wave of emotions. This facilitates using the emotional self to move in the direction of manifesting its desires. Then patterns of behavior kick in.

A keen eye is also analytical and critical at the same time, but more from the perspective of looking for opportunities to gain insights, understandings, and to exercise emotional control. When you exercise emotional control, you have that energy within your grasp to accomplish whatever it is you want. When you take that same emotional energy that could manifest as anger, resentment, frustration, agitation, or anxiety, then you harness that energy, it strengthens your control and allows you to move closer to mastery.

This is the flow of progression. You go from having an insight or an epiphany, which takes you down a path, as it should. You should be continually questioning what you are looking at, what is going on, and why it is going on. That process leads to other answers so that you eventually come to a place of understanding, which aids in emotional control, which then leads to mastery in all situations.

The keen eye may actuate, utilize, and accentuate your spiritual gifts, such as Clairvoyance, Astral Projection, and Levitation. With a keen eye, you can develop the gift of Retrocognition and Precognition, which is the ability to "look back in order to see ahead" (a Universal Teaching).

The Clinical Eye

This clinical eye looks at things differently than the keen eye. Of course, there are common elements; however, the clinical eye is more specific in what it seeks to see and understand. As an example, a particular event or experiment is created that has certain preset parameters.

An example would be drug testing. In this scenario, researchers take two groups of people and give one group the drug and the other a placebo. Everyone in the study is seen by a doctor for continual evaluation and notes are kept. At the end of the study, analytics are performed and the results are published. It is through a very similar perspective that a person observes others. This is done to gain knowledge primarily to grow the Self more than anything else. What the eyes see the mind records.

Our earliest observations were of Mom and Dad. We observed how they did things. How they were. We learned by observing, which is why some children/people seek approval as a form of acceptance. The other group choose rejection as its form of acceptance. Both work. Learn to discern what method you use so that you can begin to get a handle on it. As you do, there will be less turmoil or *dis*, allowing more peace within to manifest.

The Judgmental Eye

This is a particular perspective that some people take, which is to find something that is wrong. Once discovered, they will voice some sort of criticism about something on some level. This is a person who is unhappy in some arena of their life and feels the need to point out weaknesses or vulnerabilities in other people. When this is done, it is a way of gaining control over someone. The judgmental eye is a very critical perspective. There is the old cliché about seeing what you want to see. If the person is intent on finding fault with something, they will. No matter how mundane or minuscule the mistake (real or perceived) may be, they will find fault with it because it satisfies an internal need they have.

Keep in mind that sometimes you see what you want to see, and because you see it the way you want to see it, you will interpret it in the way that suits what you are trying to achieve, rationalize, or justify. Instead of fault-finding, aim for clarity.

Enhancing Observation

One of the ways to enhance your ability to observe is to train yourself to become sign/symbol conscious. As I mentioned earlier, symbols are something that you have already created for yourself. It is not someone else giving you a symbol, such as math symbols (+ - $ = %). Math symbols were presented to you in school, and they told you that the plus sign means to add the numbers together, and the minus sign means to subtract. Traffic signs, symbols, and lights are other forms of communication, providing guidance and awareness while you are driving.

Your mind provides you with that same type of guidance in the form of the universal perspective and your personal language, which is based on past emotional experiences. With every past emotional experience, you have an association, like your grandmother's chocolate chip cookies.

Here is another example of a personal symbol of mine. Cops on motorcycles, and police cars in general. On my way to work one morning as I was taking the off-ramp from the expressway, I saw a policeman on a motorcycle. He caught my eye for more than just a glance. I seemed to have focused on him for more than a few seconds. When I got to work five minutes later, the police, the Texas FDA, the federal FDA, the ATF, and the postal authority agents were at my business with a camera crew. It was a raid! The police had their guns drawn. They made my warehouse people get down on their knees and place their hands over their heads—just like you see in the movies.

Long story short, an employee I had fired contacted the federal authorities and falsely claimed we were selling drugs and guns. The next day, my previous boss called and said, "I don't want to wake up in the morning and see your face on national TV!" Yep, I made national news. It's not every day they can "bust" a supplement company. I eventually resolved all accusations, and it was both exhausting and a lesson in human nature (the former employee engaging in an act of retaliation) and symbolism. To this day, whenever I see a police car or motorcycle cop, I immediately start questioning, "Where am I headed? Why am I drawing authority to me? How am I moving forward and drawing authority to stop myself?"

The reason I ask the last question is because I know from past experience that the authorities can shut me down and block my forward movement, without just cause. I have confirmation that we are now prepared for an FDA, Texas, or OSHA inspection.

That is how your mind talks to you. It will give you symbols that you can relate to. However, because you have never been taught how to become symbol conscious or to read or interpret signs/symbols, your life continues on its cyclic, patternistic way. This is your personal history repeating.

The Discipline of Observation will allow you to gain control over those things observed that would have a tendency to stimulate a particular concept in your subconscious mind. Once stimulated, that concept will set in motion a particular pattern of behavior, thus creating a particular outcome. The goal in life is to create outcomes that you want; not the ones that happen from patternistic behavior.

As you become symbol conscious, you may want to get a little notebook to record what it is that your mind drew your attention to that day or hour. Then question it. Some guidance that may help you can be found in my book *The Dream Symbology Dictionary* where I have compiled a universal perspective of the symbology of many common things. There are three types of definitions for signs and symbols. First, there is a universal definition, meaning that this is an application or perspective that could pertain to everyone. However, what is more important than a universal perspective is the PEA (Personal Emotional Association) you have with a given symbol.

The third and last perspective is to look at a symbol as either positive or negative. For those who go through life with rose-colored glasses, that is the biggest mistake and the greatest trap anyone can walk into. When you have rose-colored glasses, everything is wonderful and beautiful, which only sets you up for disappointment and damage.

An aspect of observation that seems to be seldom thought about is seeking to be objective enough to be able to observe yourself in transactions. It is difficult to do; however, there is a spiritual gift called Astral Projection that allows you to get out and above yourself to observe what you are doing.

There is also another spiritual gift called Clairvoyance, which allows you to see clearly the thoughts and energies at work. There is an instantaneous "knowing" of the energy of what appears to be in front of you. There is a Universal Teaching about this ability: "Jesus said: Know what is in thy sight and what is hidden from thee will be revealed to thee. For there is nothing hidden which will not be made manifest" (*The Gospel According to Thomas* 5). Clairvoyance is also seeing everything at a glance without needing the time to do a symbolic analysis.

Another aspect of observation pertains to the imagination, which could be tied into Clairvoyance to a degree. Your imagination is you creating something in your mind's eye. These are visual images that you are creating and seeing, and maybe even responding to. The ability to look back in order to see ahead is another aspect of observation. It is based on two spiritual gifts we each possess: Retro-cognition and Precognition. From this point of view, you are using your memory to look back into the past to see how you responded or acted in a particular situation or environment. When you apply looking back to a current pattern, it is easy to see ahead how that pattern is going to complete itself. This, too, is in keeping with the Universal Teaching found in Ecclesiastes 3:15.

Observation is one of the key disciplines to be mastered. When you know what you are looking at, then you know what you are dealing with. When you can see the thought and energy behind what is taking place, it puts you in a position of strength and power. Life doesn't get any better when you possess personal power and quiet strength because that is substance; that is real. This is a power and strength that cannot be taken away from you. You cannot lose it like money or possessions or a title. The more that you grow them and the more you use them, the stronger they become.

Here are Universal Teachings that relate to observation: "The mote in your brother's eye" (Matthew 7:3), or, as stated in *The Gospel According to Thomas* 5, "Jesus said: Know what is in thy sight and what is hidden from thee will be revealed to thee. For there is nothing hidden which will not be manifest."

The Discipline of Listening

Listening is another great way of gathering knowledge and information. When you are in communication with another human being, they are telling you things about themself or things they want you to know, for one reason or another. The way you can understand the person you are dealing with, working with, or listening to is to truly listen to what is being said. It is not only the words; it's the attitude, the tone, and the implication. You are listening and observing at the same time. Listening will provide you with deeper insights.

What you hear and see on the surface is just that—surface. You have to train yourself to go deeper. What you hear does not necessarily mean that what was being said is what you received. This is because of the definitions of words. For example: "I know you heard what I said; however, that does not mean that you understood what I meant." You may say a word and I hear the word, but for me it has a completely different meaning. However, you think of it with your meaning, and I miss what you are saying. So listening is an artform and one of your spiritual gifts called Clairaudience, or Clear Hearing.

The beauty of listening to others is that you will know when someone is saying something to you that is going to trigger you. Assuming that you are on the path of self-knowledge and becoming more symbol-conscious, then you know to pay attention to what people say to you. By listening intently, the statement will not slip past your awareness and stimulate a concept and its pattern of behavior. All patterns of behavior work under the same motivation. Therefore a pattern could manifest in any number of ways. Just look at life and you can see where anger leads to difficulty, damage, and, in the extreme, death.

You are already listening to everything around you: people, music, and news. The one person you may not be listening to is yourself. People will say that they hear the small, quiet voice in their head, but they may not pay attention to it. They hear it and listen every now and then; however, that is not the best use of divine instruction and guidance, which offers you suggestions, direction, and provides input. Everything needs to be questioned. Why? Because your thoughts could be coming from an ego weighed down with doubt. Or it could be coming from your Spiritual Self, infused with inspiration. You have to decipher where the voice is coming from by being honest with Self and performing an internal examination. When you do negative self-talk, you can catch it immediately and know that you are indulging in it. Look for that quiet, still voice of strength, and let that be your guidance.

The Discipline of Sensing

This discipline incorporates the senses of taste and smell. These senses are both defensive and protective. The sense of smell can help you to avoid eating spoiled food, or it can protect you from dangerous situations such as a gas leak. I personally experienced this recently after using a new outdoor gas grill for the first time. It had an extra burner that I did not have on the old grill, and I never checked to see if it was open or closed. It wasn't until the following day while I was sitting outside enjoying the sound of chirping birds that I smelled propane. When I checked the grill, that extra burner wasn't turned off. The knob was set on low. It caused the loss of most of the propane. But if I hadn't been able to smell it, it could have caused serious damage, such as injuries or an explosion.

This demonstrates a way your senses aid you, helping you understand what energies are at work. Using the smell aspect of your senses allows you to have a handle on what is going on and how to protect yourself from what is taking place. There is a cliche that says "something smells rotten," and this does not always mean a physical substance. It is often said in regards to a situation or a statement made by someone about the "energy of the person or situation."

The Sense of Taste

You wouldn't think that the sense of taste would require a disciplined approach to living, but it does. You are tasting things when you eat. If the food was rotten and it passed your sense of smell, it may not pass your taste buds. They are there to protect you from ingesting that which could harm you. The catch-22 is that you may not be able to taste if the food is bad or not. Neither can you symbolically taste the truth of something. Whether it is good or bad for you.

The reason I phrase it that way is very simple. In our dietary habits in America, we will eat anything that is salty or sweet, even if it is bad for us. We have been conditioned to like salty and/or sweet food. An item could be rotten to the core and we might not know to stay away from it. If carbon dioxide was not used to preserve meat and give it a fresh red color, it would look like a gray piece of flesh, and you would not even consider consuming it. When something is bad, you have to be able to discern it. If not, you could consume something very harmful to your life.

Your five senses—sight, sound, taste, touch, and smell—are designed to protect and help you sort out the truth of things. You have to be able to taste the truth when someone presents an idea to you. If you don't, you could end up buying into an unrealistic approach or an unrealistic proposition, which could end up costing you dearly.

One of the spiritual gifts tied into sensing is called Psychometry, which means that you are feeling and sensing the energy of something. On another level, it is like instantly reading a sign/symbol in the Discipline of Observation and knowing immediately what is being communicated. It is an intuitive knowing and is likened to the discipline of sensing.

The Discipline of Touch

You would not think there would be such a thing as a discipline connected to touch because touch is touch. There are two ways that we touch things: physically and emotionally. Sometimes you can touch someone and inspire, motivate, and support them with your words and energy. This is a form of emotional touch. Emotional touch is what needs to be disciplined because inasmuch as you can use it as a tool for inspiration, motivation, and support, the exact opposite is also true.

You have seen the example of someone placing a finger on a person's chest and pushing them back. Energetically, the same thing can take place from an attitude that is presented to someone by pushing them away. It touches them emotionally, whether stimulating their inadequacies or their fears. But you do touch them emotionally. We all touch each other. That is why sometimes you walk into a room and there is a "knowing." Knowing if you are welcomed or not. There are some situations where you feel the energy is either welcoming or rejecting.

Overall, you may feel or think that it is going to take a lot of effort to get into a conversation with any of these people. They all know each other and seem to have an energetic relationship with one another, and you are the new energy being brought into the situation. You can sense that. You are being touched. In turn, you are reaching out to touch and feel and on a one-on-one level.

The Discipline of Speaking

Speaking is a form of communication and expression. Our words can be used as a helpful tool or a cruel weapon. They can hurt someone emotionally, or they can stir up anger. Words are incredibly powerful and trigger many different emotions. This is why it is vital that, along with the Discipline of Listening, you become mindful of what you say. Learn to control the things your speech so that you do not belittle, denigrate, attack, or raise someone's defenses. There is a Universal Teaching about this spoken by Jesus in *The Gospel According to Thomas* 14: "Jesus said: For what goes into your mouths will not defile you, but what comes out of your mouth, that is what will defile you."

You would benefit from examining your language. Record yourself so you hear how you speak and how others might hear what you are saying and how you are saying it. This would be a good exercise. When you speak, it stems from your different Selves. There is spiritual, emotional, and social speech. In spiritual speech, there are certain words in every dogma that people will relate to, and they become a normal part of conversation because it is the language of that Self and that group. A few examples are "Praise the Lord!" or "God provides!" and "The universe provides!" Each self has words that are usually germane to that self.

Discover what it is that you say repetitively, whether positive or negative. Seek to understand why you say that, then begin to exercise control over your speech. One of the ways to do this is through the Discipline of Observation by looking for symbols—things that you know will trigger you or will seek to stimulate the concept that will trigger the pattern.

The more mindful and disciplined you are, the greater control you will have over yourself, which is truly the only thing you can control. From this point of personal power, you know that your energy is centered and focused, and there is no one and nothing that can disrupt it.

The Discipline of Health

Health is a multiple book topic. In fact, there are thousands of books written on the subject. I have written one called *The Naturopathic Healing Handbook*, which is a nutritional approach to healing. Another book I have written is an examination of health conditions from an emotional and symbolic point of view called *The Emotional Causes of Disease*, which contains over seventy diseases and covers multiple health matters, including how accidents are related to diseases. Nutritional guidance is also provided, as well the emotional significance of diet. The information given helps you see and understand why the need exists for certain nutrients, in high potency, to help bring the body back to balance and harmony.

Disease symbolically represents an emotional conflict taking place subconsciously. It is the conflict centered on being who you think you should be contrasted against who it is you want to be. There may also be conflicting energy surrounding who you think you need to be. Ultimately, the goal is to have your Spiritual Self be the dominate Self, not the Emotional Self.

When it comes to the Discipline of Health, obviously the first matter you need to examine is your diet. What does is it consist of? Which category would you consider yourself to be in? Do you have a diet that favors being a carnivore, lacto-ovo vegetarian, vegetarian, vegan, fruitarian, or strictly raw food?

What are you consuming in the way of beverages? Sodas, juices, water, or alcohol? Each have aspects that require considerations. For instance, soda can create osteoporosis because of the phosphoric acid, which carries calcium out of the body. Juices may have too much sugar, possibly leading to weight gain if there isn't enough exercise to burn off the calories.

When it comes to water, I am a distilled water advocate. You don't know where the water has been. It could have flowed under a nuclear power facility or paper manufacturing plant. There's no telling. With distilled water, I feel "better safe than sorry." To me, the body represents many things. In this presentation, it's about the body's health. The healthier the diet, the healthier the body. The reward? A slower aging process.

One example of the body is to view it as an orchestra, each gland, system, organ, and function representing a particular section of the orchestra. In order for a classical piece to be played, each instrument has to be in tune. Together, all of those instruments create a beautifully harmonious sound.

However, if strings on one of the instruments break, and somebody's reed from the wind section cracks, the notes they are going to play will be a little out of harmony. This would be comparable to only one cell being out of harmony, and therein lies the beginning of physical aging and corruption.

In terms of the body, poor health (such as colds, flu, and various diseases) can occur because of being malnourished. In this state, it is susceptible to attack or malformation upon cell division, which is naturally occurring. This will lead to conditions and diseases as it multiplies. However, illness can be slowed, stopped from progressing, or eliminated completely.

Poor health conditions multiply through an imbalanced and nutritionally weak body. So what corrects this situation? Diet, exercise, and supplementation. From experience, that equates to investing in high-potency supplements. A good mindset rounds out the fundamentals.

There is a spiritual gift associated with health: Healing. There are three parts to Healing: faith, belief, and expectation.

Faith, Belief, and Expectation

Here's an example of how it works. You may have heard that a certain doctor, naturopath, herbalist, chiropractor, or masseuse is really fabulous, and if you will work with them, they will fix whatever is wrong and you will feel great. You call and make the appointment to see them. You walked in there with "faith" at work. Now the practitioner has spent some time with you, and upon leaving you're given a prescription and a list of recommendations or suggestions. Now, "belief" is going to work.

In your hand sits the prescription, or the practitioner's suggestions. You go to the drug store or the health food store because you want to get the recommended products so you feel better. The "expectation" is that once you get ahold of everything (meds, vitamins, herbs, minerals, foods, juices) and start taking them, they will make you feel great. Your "expectation" is at work here.

Goal-Seeking

Your mind is a goal-seeking, goal-driven biocomputer that uses the energy of expectation through patterns of behavior to accomplish its goals. The primary purpose is proving the subconscious concept that was stimulated as being true. Patterns are the software program, and expectations are the energies that run them until complete. In essence, you live to fulfill expectations on all levels. Part of that is because expectations validate a subconscious concept that you maintain about yourself.

This is why you can change patterns of behavior, because there is an expectation of a particular type of result at the end. Knowing that gives you the opportunity to change it completely, creating a different result. In this application, it would be healing on another level.

Consider that your body is a temple. This was expressed by Jesus when he taught that the "kingdom is within." "Neither shall they say, Lo here! or, Lo there! For, behold, the Kingdom of God is within you" (Luke 17:21). The example of Jesus chasing the money changers out of the temple courtyard is symbolic of him cleaning up the temple. This is why it is essential to attain good health. You have to clean up your body. It is taught that the body is a spiritual, holy temple. Re-examine your dietary choices. Your health, vitality, and life are up to you. Feed yourself well on all levels.

The Doctrine of Personal Responsibility

The Doctrine of Personal Responsibility is based on the understanding that everything that takes place in your life is the result of your co-creation. You participated in creating it because it fulfills a concept in your subconscious mind. You create specific patterns of behavior with a drive to achieve a particular result. The result is generated through the energy of expectation. You are always seeking to fulfill expectations because they continually validate your subconscious concepts, such as being who you think you are supposed to be. You alone are creating the life you are living.

Your life is a reflection of the subconscious concepts you maintain. These concepts you have accepted as true and necessary are designed to provide you with a mode of acceptance. The acceptance is from your mother. The reason being is it is through her, the birth canal, you entered into the material plane, physical reality. Each of us is a spiritual being in a material body. Each of us at a deep subconscious level wants to go "home" because we know this world we live in is insane. We believe as long as we have Mom's acceptance, we are guaranteed a way back to the spiritual plane, a place of peace and tranquility.

Acceptance from Mom comes in two forms. One of which you are currently manifesting. The two forms of acceptance are approval and rejection. Either of these is based on many factors, such as your mother wanting or not wanting to be pregnant; another could be her experiencing an easy or difficult pregnancy. As you can see by the doctrine, ultimately you are 100 percent responsible for everything that unfolds in your life. Even when someone else is involved, they, too, are 100 percent responsible because nothing happens by itself.

Whatever thought you have, whatever thinking is stimulated by that thought, whatever action is taken based on that, it all stems from you. You are the Creator. It doesn't matter if someone triggers you into any type of emotional reaction, such as anger or resentment. You are still responsible based on two perspectives: The first perspective is your reaction. This must be controlled. The second perspective is to ask yourself, "Why did I draw that to me?"

Here is one more reason why you must read sign and symbols and develop eyes to see and ears to hear. When someone says something to you or makes a facial gesture, you know instantaneously that it has the potential to create a disturbance within you on some level. Know that you will ultimately be responsible for the way things unfold. So no matter what takes place, you are ultimately responsible.

When the Doctrine of Personal Responsibility becomes a habit, you become a living example of that discipline. You first become a disciple unto the concept of personal responsibility, then you become a spiritual teacher—a living example of what it means to be a responsible human being, exemplifying the Doctrine of Personal Responsibility.

Here is your personal doctrine: *I am responsible for everything that happens to me. I created the situation to bring about the result. I set in motion the situations, events, and thoughts that will culminate in a particular way to create a particular event. I am constantly co-creating my reality to validate my subconscious concepts of who I think I should be.*

I know that I am co-creating my reality with the Creative Continuum called God.

The Discipline of Unity

What is unity? What does it mean? Here are a few definitions I gleaned from Wiktionary: "oneness; the state or fact of being one undivided entity; single thing, seen as complete in itself." These are good definitions; however, for our purposes there are two types of unity that need to be examined: the unity that exists externally, such as demonstrated in an athletic team, and the unity that exists within the Self. This is the unity of male and female, spiritual and physical energies.

The question to ask is, "What is within that must be unified?" Since you are a spiritual being encased in a material body, your "vehicle" must be in balance and harmony within. Additionally, you are both male and female. These two must also be unified. Both gender hormones exist in your body, so you could say, from a symbolic point of view, that although you are a male, you would have empathy and other aspects as a female would. On the other hand, as a female you would have elements and aspects of expression as a male might.

Another very important type of unity is exemplified in a relationship. The key components to a good relationship/partnership are respect for the other person, good communication, enjoying the other person's company, and, above all, *love*. An aspect of this unity ties into the Doctrine of Personal Responsibility expressed below. In that, you are 100 percent responsible for whatever takes place in your life. This also includes the truth that whatever happens to the other person in your intimate relationship, you had a part in its occurrence.

Of course, there are hereditary and genetic situations that you did not participate in creating. In this situation, the concepts involved need to be examined by both parties. This should open a series of questions, which is a good thing because answers will provide insights. Insights lead to understandings. Understandings, in turn, lead to control and mastery. The control that must be exercised is emotional.

Unity without is a reflection of unity within. How does one achieve this unity within? You have spiritual gifts that can help you with that task. One gift is Telepathy and another is Levitation. These are both connected to unity.

Telepathy is a matter of opening up your mind to communicate within and without through thought. In order for that to occur, there has to be the elimination of defenses and complete control over your thinking process. In being telepathic, a person is also wide open. This implies nondefensiveness. Some couples have Telepathy between one another because it is an energetic form of communication. Many times you and your partner will say the same thing at the same moment in the same way. Or you may say, "I just had that thought" when your partner brings up a topic.

With training, Telepathy can be developed to perform at higher and deeper levels. Here are examples of what I used to do as a salesman when presenting a new product. If there was a person in the store who was talking and talking to the owner without saying anything of value (I know you know people like that), I would stand a few feet behind them and project the thought, *I have to go home now*, over and over. In a matter of moments the person would say, "I have to go home now," then leave. Now I had the owner to myself. Another way I would use telepathy was to "tell" the retailer to "expand the line" on the store shelves, since I represented a very good supplement line.

The spiritual gift of Levitation allows you to walk on water, so to speak. Walking on water as demonstrated by Jesus and Peter is symbolic of mastering the material plane. You walk above the material so that you are not immersed in it. It would be like walking on a concrete floor versus walking on sand. On sand, your toes will sink down, slowing your forward movement. If the sand is very wet, it could hold you down. On concrete, you are solidly on top of it and free to roam. From this solid footing, you understand that you are here to master the material plane on multiple levels. Being above it releases you from it.

The freer you can be, the higher you can Levitate your mind, your spirit, and— eventually—your body. When you have a deeper understanding of your Self and the energy flow of Earth's gravity, you will be able to manipulate the energy to serve you. There are ethereal energies as well that one needs to master in order to be able to Levitate. By exercising discipline in any area of your life, you will have positive growth benefits. Guaranteed.

The Twelve Spiritual Gifts

Man has been endowed with twelve spiritual gifts to help him master his life and the material plane and restore balance and harmony.

- Understanding
- Knowledge
- Expression
- Imagination
- Will
- Perseverance
- Faith
- Strength
- Objectivity
- Honesty
- Healing
- Love

Understanding

When you hear and use the word and concept of understanding, you say you understand this or that. You rarely think of the definition of the word *understand*, so here are a few synonyms to contemplate:

- Comprehension
- Intelligence
- Good sense
- Discernment
- Compassion
- Sympathy
- The ability to learn, judge, or make decisions

You know and understand some things and not others. When it comes to the Self, you may only know or understand a limited amount of information as to the whys and wherefores of how and what you think. Even within the concept of understanding, there are very distinct levels. For instance, there are the basic understandings that affect life, such as the understanding that you require food, water, and air to exist.

Understandings are essential to successful living on the emotional, social, physical/material, and spiritual levels. Developing the depth of your own understandings and discovering new ones will lead to mastery of your life in greater degrees than you are experiencing now.

A fundamental understanding is of how *reality itself* is created. As you know, atoms are the fundamental building blocks of material reality. With either a positive or a negative charge, they bind together, based on attraction, to create molecules that grow and become the substance of every type and description of physical entity that you can think of, including living human beings.

Water has three states of matter: solid, liquid, or gas. In its liquid state, it can condense into ice or it can expand into gas. As the temperature goes down, the vibratory energy of the atoms begins to slow, and they condense and solidify. In the opposite state, heat expands the atoms. Atoms can be looked at from a symbolic point of view, keeping in mind the fundamental understanding that everything is created out of atoms. Another amazing fundamental understanding is that the brain is an electromagnetic generator; in fact, there is a patent[8] for a device for measuring brain and heart electromagnetic waves. Most people are unaware of this attribute of the mind/brain combination. This is an incredible piece of information to help you understand how you are co-creating your reality and how the Universal Teaching of "ask and you shall receive" works. The catch is that you must be in control of your subconscious desires and "askings" to have true control over your manifestations.

As an electromagnetic generator operated by your mind, your brain is either sending out positive, attracting energy waves (electromagnetic waves) or repulsive electromagnetic waves. Just like a magnet, it repels and attracts. When you take in both understandings, that of the atomic makeup of the material world and the electromagnetic generating potential of the mind/brain, and utilize that knowledge, you can create the reality that you desire. Your current personal reality is that of electromagnetically drawing to yourself energy whose atoms and molecules are manifesting as a person, place, and/or event. On the same note, you may be repelling energetic combinations manifesting as a person or thing, such as success or money. The questions to ask here are: "What am I attracting?" and "What am I keeping away from me?" I choose the words

---

[8] U.S. Patent #5,307807

"keeping away" because they imply more than repelling. There are some energy manifestations that you want in your life, yet you do not have them. One such example may be having a companion. For instance, you might have developed socially unacceptable habits as a safety mechanism to repel people from getting close. Through the process of understanding, you can attract or keep away specific energies.

When you understand the influences (energies) behind the motivations that propel you to take certain actions, you can exercise control over those emotional directives and their responses. Control is one of the main tools in the mastery of Self. It is through understanding your concepts that operate in the subconscious and then exercising emotional influence over your patterns of behavior that you are able to significantly change your life.

Here is an example of how negative energy was affecting my business, and how we revolved it. My company has sales cycles. There are days when business is brisk and days when it is slow. Although our phones usually ring all day on Mondays, I noticed one Monday the phones were relatively silent. I realized the usual flow of energy was blocked like a dam blocking a river.

I began questioning myself as well as seeking to understand the energy of the crew. I brought this to the attention of my general manager, and she informed me there was an issue between a couple of the employees. Once I understood the situation, I had a meeting with all parties involved. We discussed different perspectives and understandings of the issue, and it was resolved (as communication commonly achieves), and the energy was restored to normal. Everyone understood the situation and their attitudes changed, thereby changing the energy of the office. Almost immediately, the phones began to ring off the hook.

In my own personal reflections, I was able to see how I helped create the negative situation as well. In all of our involvements, we are 100 percent responsible. The goal is to understand and master Self and cleanse man-made concepts from our minds. As you gain insights that lead to understandings, you will have a greater degree of self-acceptance, allowing more of the God Energy within you to manifest. You can allow Divine Grace as the channel for Divine Love to manifest in everything that you do—for the sake of tranquility, for the sake of unity, and for the sake of man-made convention. By understanding why you are attracted to the people you are attracted to, why you act the way that you do, and why you are afraid to act differently, you can attain a great base of power.

Operating on the concept of sacrifice, some folks always do what they consider to be the right thing, even if it is detrimental to Self. They often take actions and maintain attitudes that are not conducive to growth. Sometimes they indulge in denial of Self because they think it is the right thing to do in man-made, conventional terms. The only way to break out of man-made conventional concepts is to understand the Universal Truths. In striving to reach that level of understanding and manifest it in your life, it may mean that you come into conflict with everything in your embedded belief system and with everyone who is a part of your life. If others are not willing to move in the same direction as you at the same time, then you have major issues. Here is where you realize that you may be on separate paths.

You may be in a relationship and a unity that has lasted many years, and one day you realize that the two of you are on different tracks, have different needs and desires, and that your path of enlightenment has taken you one place and your partner's path is directed elsewhere. Who is right and who is wrong? Is there a right and a wrong? It all comes down to understanding yourself, your needs, and your quest to fulfill your needs based on Universal Truth.

During one of the various study group meetings that I present, one of the participants asked, "Based on what you said about different paths, if you understand yourself, you won't find yourself in a relationship where your path of enlightenment is separate from the other. So is it possible to be in a relationship where both are not on the same track? With the same needs, desires, and paths of enlightenment?"

I answered, "I know that there is an expression that opposites attract; however, that is in magnetism and not necessarily true for all people. We are driven by our subconscious concepts. When it comes to a partner, there are many things that come into consideration, especially spiritual beliefs. There must be enough commonality between the two individuals for it to work. A Universal Teaching reflecting this is, "A divided house cannot stand[9]"

Can different relationships with different individuals at different times be stepping-stones to enlightenment? It sure seems that way. As we go through life, we meet those who can teach, guide, and inspire us. When we get to a certain age and think we know it all, that is when the trouble begins.

---

[9] "And Jesus knew their thoughts, and said unto them, Every kingdom divided against itself is brought to desolation; and every city or house divided against itself shall not stand.—"Matthew 12:25

Another aspect to the answer lies in the concept of true unity. At some point there would be mental telepathy, because there would no longer be any defenses at work, an accomplishment that takes decades, if not lifetimes, to achieve. Going through relationship after relationship is an indicator of a misconception at work. "Wouldn't all relationships between individuals seeking to fulfill needs based on Universal Truth be on the same path?" someone else asked, to which I replied, "In essence, yes."

Another question: "Are there other types of directives besides emotional ones?" The answer simply is no. It is the Emotional Self, the ego, that seeks to manifest in everything that it is doing. This is the aspect of Self that is the fundamental director of the physical, material, and social self.

Knowledge

Knowledge and understanding are synonymous with each other. Understanding is your stable foundation based upon the knowledge accumulated through education and life experiences. Knowledge is more fluid than understanding and provides many ways that it can be employed. Also, knowledge is a "knowing," a sensing of things, people, situations, and events.

A good example is when you walk into a room and you immediately "sense" the energy. Similarly, you can have an instant attraction to someone based on energetic exchanges at a "knowing or sensing" level. Another example is thinking a certain person was going to call and moments later the phone rings and it is the very person you had in mind. Knowledge is a foundational stepping-stone to understanding. The more you know about something, the more apt you are to grow and gain a deeper understanding of the matter. The stronger your desire is to know and understand something, the greater the rewards of that effort.

How do you gain knowledge? Of course, the easy answer is schooling, which is a way of learning and thinking that is not necessarily in a person's best interest. In the acquisition of knowledge, do not confuse it with intellect; many people understand something intellectually yet cannot apply it. You see this in religions and areas of faith, complete with rituals. If you cannot apply the information and improve your life, then it doesn't work. With no fundamental essence other than acceptance, you are indulging in blind faith as opposed to a working faith.[10] Be clear about the difference between true self-knowledge and intellectual knowledge, between man-made understandings and Universal Teachings. For instance, from a man-made point of view, the male is the dominant partner, the provider and protector. However, in Genesis, there is the Universal Teaching addressing the roles of the sexes: male and female are equal.[11] Eve being created out of the rib of Adam is a symbolic metaphor indicating that the female aspect of Self is part of the protection system, the ribcage, and it protects your innards. The female aspect is a source of inner strength because it's made from bone, which is your support system and "inner strength. "

The intellect can trick us. Look around and you can see that it has, in the sense of our technological age. We have a wonderful life, while at the same time, technology is poisoning us with many chemicals in the environment that corrupt cells that contribute greatly to the aging process and to diseases such as cancer. We are paying for our modern technological life with our health.

Another intellectual pursuit is marketing, which is conditioning you to follow a particular diet or to buy a particular food. Education, on the other hand, is more valuable because the knowledge that it supplies comes from so many different sources. The most important knowledge that is essential for a balanced and prosperous life is that of the Self, your Self.

One important method for gaining self-knowledge is to listen to what you say. Listen to how you speak—the tone, the veracity, the velocity, and the essential energy behind it. Once you can hear yourself, you will also have an insight into how others hear you. Listen to your choices of words. Are they inspiring or debilitating? If and when you find yourself in negative thinking, speaking, or reacting, ask yourself, "Why does this bother me? What is behind these feelings?"

Expression
Like understanding and knowledge, expression seems to be a common, everyday thing, something that everyone uses to some degree. You would not think of such an everyday

---

[10] A working faith is built on understanding, experience and knowing that whatever you are confronted with, you can handle it.

[11] "So God created man in his own image, in the **image** of God created he him; male and female created he them." —Genesis 1:27

quality as a spiritual gift, and yet it is, along with others that you will discover as you continue to go through this process of examination.

Expression is a vehicle that takes you places. On one level, you say automatically, "Of course I express myself. I talk every day. I interact with people, and I'm a social being. I have a special type of a job. That, too, is a form of expression." Yes, that is all true, and there are other forms of expression. You may be someone who enjoys the arts. You may even paint, write, play music, or sculpt. All of these are different forms of expression, each with its own unique nuances as well as the discipline to create the final form. Other forms of expression may be engineering, mechanics, or sales. Expression is one of the ways in which a person can influence others and present himself to the world. In encounters, you display one or more of the four aspects of Self (spiritual, emotional, social, and physical/material), depending upon with whom you are interacting and the associated concepts that are triggered. The stimuli and symbols that are presented will determine from where you will respond.

The Emotional Self is the most fruitful ground to explore to enhance your expression because it directly relates to your subconscious concepts and belief system. All reactions evolve out of the Emotional Self foundation and influence your actions in the social, spiritual, and the physical/material Self. I always say physical/material because I would have you think about your physical body as the physical aspect of Self and your material reality as a manifestation of your entire essence. If you are a billionaire, a "dollaraire," or anywhere in between, all of that is in keeping with concepts, patterns, and expectations, which is how your material reality is formed. This is a reflection of the Universal Teaching: "What is within will manifest without."

Question your expression and how you use it in each arena of your life. By understanding how you express yourself, you will be able to appreciate, from a different point of view, how others express themselves. Seek to understand how some forms of expression trigger you in a positive or negative way. I really do not like to use the terms "positive" and "negative," yet when you become aware of something that stimulates your patterns or triggers a concept, you will see why it is in your best interest to develop a symbol dictionary. Expression is an extension of Self and a developed sense of feeling and of being. By understanding expression, you will be able to intuitively assess the energy of a situation.

Imagination

Imagination is a wonderful thing, and it is unfortunate when someone is taught, "Do not waste your time in daydreaming, imagining, or wishful thinking." The imagination is a direct link to tomorrow, to the future. Many of today's technical marvels had their beginnings in science fiction stories and movies from decades past. Maybe you have had this experience: You get an idea, yet you do not have the resources to pursue it on your own. You may present a good idea to your company, with no takers, and then a short time later your idea manifests in another company. Sometimes the ideas that emanate from your imagination end up being capitalized upon by others.

One way I often describe how imagination is used to think up a new idea is to compare it with going fishing. Ideas are like fish in a stream, and fish are symbolic of thoughts. The Creative Continuum's Supreme Consciousness is an ocean of God. As soon as you have an idea and pull it out of the stream of consciousness, once you start thinking about it, toying with it and discussing it, the idea is now available to others. This is a concept is similar to the "100 monkey" theory. The story is that a monkey found a sweet potato that was very sandy, so she went down to the water to wash it off. She did that every day until a couple of other monkeys saw her do this, and they started doing it. When 100 monkeys were seen washing their food before eating it, all the monkeys of the tribe did it, and monkeys on neighbor islands did it. Eventually, monkeys around the world began washing their food.[12] At a certain level or vibration, an idea becomes public domain, available to all who think and seek.

Your imagination can take you to wonderful places. Developing it takes practice. Pick a topic, an area, an endeavor, a dream, or a vacation spot. The more you can imagine yourself there, the more real you can make it, and the energy necessary to create that reality will ultimately manifest because you are "asking" consciously. Inasmuch as you bring an idea into the material plane, so can somebody else, and you may be picking up on an idea that they did not manifest. Once you come upon an idea, run with it. Do not hesitate, whether it's yours or theirs, because the first one to market is the winner.

Look at the science fiction novels and comic books of years ago. Gadgets today are almost up to Dick Tracy's wristwatch videophone—today we have desktops, laptops, iPods, and smartphones. Someone's imagination many decades ago pulled that idea out of the ocean, and it eventually entered the material plane. The gadget was presented as an idea, and that idea bore fruit. That cartoonist saw the future—look at Star Trek and the paperless technology. Maybe the iPad is what Captain Kirk used. So develop your imagination and see where it can take you. Use your mind in a new, inventive way. Stretch it to look at something and alter it, or create a new way of using it.

----

[12] *The Hundredth Monkey* by Ken Keyes, Jr.

The Japanese monkey, Macaca Fuscata, had been observed in the wild for a period of over thirty years. In 1952, on the island of Koshima, scientists were providing monkeys with sweet potatoes dropped in the sand. The monkeys' liked the taste of the raw sweet potatoes, but they found the dirt unpleasant. An eighteen-month-old female named Imo found she could solve the problem by washing the potatoes in a nearby stream. She taught this trick to her mother. Her playmates also learned this new way and they taught their mothers too.

This cultural innovation was gradually picked up by various monkeys before the eyes of the scientists. Between 1952 and 1958 all the young monkeys learned to wash the sandy sweet potatoes to make them more palatable. Only the adults who imitated their children learned this social improvement. Other adults kept eating the dirty sweet potatoes. Then something startling took place. In the autumn of 1958, a certain number of Koshima monkeys were washing sweet potatoes—the exact number is not known. Let us suppose that when the sun rose one morning there were 99 monkeys on Koshima Island who had learned to wash their sweet potatoes. Let's further suppose that later that morning, the hundredth monkey learned to wash potatoes. THEN IT HAPPENED!

By that evening almost everyone in the tribe was washing sweet potatoes before eating them. The added energy of this hundredth monkey somehow created an ideological breakthrough! But notice. A most surprising thing observed by these scientists was that the habit of washing sweet potatoes then jumped over the sea. Colonies of monkeys on other islands and the mainland troop of monkeys at Takasakiyama began washing their sweet potatoes too. Thus, when a certain critical number achieves an awareness, this new awareness may be communicated from mind to mind.

Although the exact number may vary, this hundredth monkey phenomenon means that when only a limited number of people know of a new way, it may remain the conscious property of these people. But there is a point at which if only one more person tunes-in to a new awareness, a field is strengthened so that this awareness is picked up by almost everyone! (From the book *The Hundredth Monkey* by Ken Keyes, Jr. The book is not copyrighted and the material may be reproduced in whole or in part.)

One of the things you can use your imagination for is healing—through relaxation and meditation. When you are in those states, visualize the part of your body in disease and see it healed. Your imagination tells your brain, your biocomputer, to fix your physical situation to reflect the one that you are now projecting in your mind's eye, your imagination. Enhance the process by imagining the area bathed in red, drawing blood, or imagine a laser light eliminating the damaged tissue; the laser can be a scalpel or a suture. Finally, use your imagination to bathe the entire area in green, the color of healing.

Willpower

Willpower can make you Master of the Universe. Well, at least the master of your own reality. Every day you use willpower, the incredible gift and tool that most people never think twice about. It focuses your mental strength to manifest your intentions in everything you do, and patterns are no exceptions. Your will drives you to fulfill your subconscious expectations of yourself.

Try this exercise: Divide a blank piece of paper, and on the left side write what you believe your personality traits are and how others might see you. On the right side, write why that might be and why you may be that type of personality. See where that takes you to understand that you are using your will to fulfill expectations and those traits that help you maintain the image you have built around who you think you should be. The concepts that produce expectations are buried deep within, and discovering them helps you to gain greater control over your will so that you manifest what you, the aware one, want.

Your mind is like a biocomputer, with some programs that need to be erased, others fixed, and new ones added. With these improvements, your mind will run smoother and faster at manifesting your desires. Your Spiritual Self is seeking to manifest the will of God in everything you do to help you attain love, beauty, harmony, balance, and appropriateness in your life. As spiritual energy is trying to manifest, your Emotional Self influences it and to some degree is altered. The ability to achieve a particular end is hindered because of the Emotional Self's determination to remain the same. Remember, your Emotional Self does not want to change or to give itself up. In order for your Spiritual Self to manifest its powers more fully, you must understand the Emotional Self, which is a process. It all begins by identifying patterns of behavior and seeing the cycles as they have unfolded in the past. Seek to understand the concepts supporting your patterns and how they seek validation in a cyclical fashion; your patterns create expectations designed to validate your concepts. Once you understand them, you can exercise your will in such a way as to control the manifestations of those patterns. In this state, you can direct the outcome.

Perseverance

Every gift, like the mind itself, should be considered a muscle; if you are not using your gifts, they will become flaccid, and when they lose their tone internally, the body/mind does not function nearly as well as it could. Perseverance is a gift that needs to be strengthened and utilized.

While understanding is something you develop, knowledge is something you acquire, and expression is something you do, perseverance is something you draw on. Expression, through perseverance, demonstrates your understanding and knowledge. When you channel it through the gift of love and/or healing, things work in harmony within yourself and everyone you come in contact with. To get through the man-made concepts so you can reach the deep, internal spiritual pool of the All, take care to persevere through the internal questioning of Self, just as you persevere through difficult situations. When people give up on perseverance, they can be smashed down by life. But when you persevere with a good attitude, you have more opportunities for growth, advancement, and success. The best way to have a good attitude is knowing and understanding who you are and having clarity about everything that is going on around you. Be aware and intentional about what you are involved in and what your expression might be.

Faith

Rather than a spiritual gift, faith is a natural part of life. Faith is acceptance of Self and of God, our Father/Mother, and faith accomplishes what you set your mind to do. For many, faith is an external thing. Most people would say, "I have faith in God" or in something else. Another type of faith is internal, a faith in your Self to handle any situation. Your working faith is productive because it is built on understanding, and confidence is the outward manifestation. Understanding who you are and what you are capable of provides a solid foundation.

Every time you are confronted with a situation, your mind looks back to see how to handle it using a working faith because it is looking back to see the origin of the energy. This is where the Universal Teaching of "look back in order to see ahead" comes into play. Ask yourself: "What type of faith do I have? Where is my faith strong and where is it weak?" Are there some areas in which you have a lot of confidence in yourself—your working faith in action—when you know you can do the job and there is no question in your mind whatsoever?

There may be situations that you shy away from, either consciously or subconsciously, because you do not have faith in yourself and your ability to deal with them from a position of strength. Your doubt and fear are at work, undermining your faith in Self. The solutions lie within you if you will pursue them. Allow the insights you need to grow your understandings so that the gifts you have can help you be free of the material plane.

When you have faith in yourself, you can get through the darkest of times because you know that you are part of the Creative Continuum called God, the Father/Mother. You know that you are never placed in a situation you cannot handle, and you know that you are never alone. Regardless of how isolated you may be or feel, God is with you deep within. Draw comfort from that, and let it be a foundation of your working faith. You can also let it assist you in developing skills, methods, techniques, and understandings that enable you to become the master of your Self through the expression of faith and strength.

Strength

How do you gauge your strength? I often say, "Deal with a situation from a position of strength." Strength means being extremely confident in yourself, which is achieved when you know and understand what is going on and what energies are at work. Strength is also knowing that you have the wherewithal to move forward on a particular path; for instance, you may be strong in math and weak in biology. Seek to identify your personal strengths.

I am working with a gentleman who is quite a perfectionist and a skilled craftsman; yet he denigrates his own work and denies any compliments. If you say something nice to him, like many people, he will say, "Oh no, no, no, not me. Anybody could do that." When you do that, it is a way of depleting your strength, because by not acknowledging it, you negate it.

There is a Universal Teaching for strength: "Use what you have and more will be given; do not use what you have and it shall be taken from you." Read the story of the "Talents of Gold.[13]" Strength is like a muscle. The more you exercise and build on it, the stronger you become. Here is one exercise: Pick a project that you're working on. Let's

---

[13] Matthew 25:1429–

say that you are in the process of producing a complicated report with many components. On a piece of paper, note the weaknesses and the strengths of the report. These are things you need to keep in mind and understand because, depending upon the concepts at work at the time, your mind is going to choose one concept. Your mind is going to look back and see what is in keeping with the current situation. Which one will you draw upon, strength or weakness?

Have your mind draw on positive experiences versus unsuccessful ones, and become comfortable and familiar with your strengths, regardless of the varying degrees. Once you begin to read symbols, you can project into the future to have a feel for what will unfold and, having some alternative thoughts, you will have alternative plans of action so that you are prepared to deal with what does unfold.

Another type of strength will be developed as your understandings and knowledge base grows. As the power of your expression unfolds, you will manifest "quiet strength," the strength of knowing in action, which allows for having a nondefensive response to anything that is said to you. This strength provides inner calm and peace when things are difficult, allowing you to see with clarity when others cannot. It also exudes an energy that helps others to be at peace and wonder what your secret is.

Objectivity

The more personal and emotional the event or situation, the more difficult it is to attain objectivity. More often than not, you may feel involved because there is an emotional connection that alters your perception. With emotional involvement, you see things through your shaded belief system. Like opening your eyes under water, you have no clarity, only distorted perception.

The degree of objectivity you attain will be based on different foundations. One could be a non-emotional involvement, with no connection whatsoever, so that the outcome is immaterial to you and has no bearing on your life. The more detached you are, the more objective you can become. Jesus said, "Be passers-by.[14]" When you project yourself above the situation to look at it from as many different angles as you can, seeking clarity, then your understandings of any situation will grow immensely.

Right now there are many things for which you have feelings and attitudes. What are they? Why are they? Write your questions and answers on a sheet of paper to ponder these and the many other questions that will arise as you explore your Inner Self with

---

[14] *The Gospel According to Thomas* 42

objectivity. Write your thoughts and concerns down and place them in the conscious realm. Once you explore them consciously, you are working with your intent: "I wrote this out. I'm going to do it. I intend to get this done."

You may be the kind of person who would benefit immensely from writing down your goals and creating a plan of action to help you achieve your goals, step by step. By being objective and looking at these completely detached and unemotional, you can look at the pros and cons and do the 4 Ps (Plan, Prepare, Project, and Provide).

It is hard to be objective when people trigger your subconscious concepts through physical gestures, stances, and positions. If you are not reading your symbols and maintaining a high degree of awareness, then your patterns will be triggered and your perceptions and understandings will be affected. Your objectivity may be compromised to the degree of emotional stimulation and involvement in any given situation.

Working with and counseling a woman, I helped her through a difficult situation. She runs a company and has two subordinates, both men with whom she had issues. When looking objectively, we discovered her concepts of men and how she shaded her perceptions by her concepts and emotions. We began to see her patterns and their patterns at work. We examined how the men both had issues with authority, and with "moms" and parents in general. When you have these types of interactions going on, the best thing is to detach yourself emotionally and become a passerby. Avoid looking at things through an emotional perspective. Seek to maintain your objectivity at all times.

Learning to look at things symbolically can be helpful, as everything has an energetic thought behind it. See the object/event/person as what they may mean to you. What is your association with them? You will discover, from an objective viewpoint, that there is a connection.

Honesty

One of the most difficult things in spiritual growth is being honest with yourself. The more honest you can be with yourself, the more you are open to receive. Honesty is the result of internal questioning. In *The Gospel According to Thomas* 2, Jesus said, "Seek and ye shall find. When you *find*, you will be *troubled*. After you have *troubled*, you will *marvel* and *reign* over the All." Briefly, this simply means that if you look within yourself, you are going to think all kinds of negative things about yourself that you have been taught. However, they are not true, and that will be the marvel.

On the other hand, some of us, in our journey through life and operating patternistically, have done things to hurt other people on different levels and in different ways, more out of patterns than out of intent. Remember that patterns of behavior live and operate to reach a conclusion, to fulfill an expectation. By fulfilling the expectation, it validates the concept.

Perhaps there are horrible things that you have done to people out of seeking to fulfill a concept. Accept what you have done, examine it, and learn from it so you can move forward without guilt, understanding that what you did was based on your concepts. Once you begin to realize that life is different than you may have been taught, it opens up a whole new panorama that will assist you in your growth and the development of your abilities to understand, to know, and to express.

Honesty is something built slowly. You already have, to some degree, a second cornerstone upon which to build a new foundation and to enhance your spiritual and material expression. As events happen, look for symbols and think about why and what is going on.

Be open and honest with everyone you meet, even if that makes you feel vulnerable, which it will. The more you know about yourself, the more you come from a position of strength. Nothing anybody can say or do from the past could hurt you, embarrass you, or humiliate you. When you have understanding of Self, you will be able to control your emotional responses.

Healing

The enlightened ones of yesterday knew that the body is the healer of itself. In today's world, drugs are used to alleviate discomfort. Of course, there are antibiotics that supposedly kill germs. Yet when there is talk about diseases (like arthritis, diabetes, edema or obesity), all of these are self-correctable conditions, unless there is a severe glandular malfunction from a genetic or damaged point of view. However, if it is just because a gland is malnourished and cannot produce the proper enzymes or hormones necessary for the proper functioning of the body, that is a nutrition issue.

The body will heal itself if given what it needs. People think of healing as going to the doctor, naturopath, homeopath, or to an herbalist. While each of those may serve a purpose from time to time, you would benefit more if you were to nurture yourself back to health than to take an artificial approach. Healing is something for your physical body and your spiritual, emotional, material and social self. Healing does not necessarily imply that there is disease or sickness; it is an ongoing process because your body is in a constant state of rebuilding itself and your life is in a constant state of unfolding.

Every disease begins within the subconscious mind, in keeping with expectations, and it can also be the result of conflict. Because of the way life flows in cycles, and because of patterns of behavior that utilize those cycles, you have both forward movement and standstill (or backward) movement.

Look at each aspect of Self and see where more nutrients or nurturing are necessary. What are the nutrients? In a physical/material sense, it is about diet, exercise, vitamins, minerals, herbs, amino acids, water, air, and sunlight—the things that nurture you on a physical level.

On an emotional level, it may be an ongoing self-conversation, positive affirmations, deep meditation and prayer, connecting with God, the Creative Continuum within, and communicating your wants, needs, and desires. These are tools to help you on your path and to learn to use visions.[15] Visions are the result of using your imagination to see the areas of your body or your life that require healing. See the aspects in your social life and or spiritual life that would benefit from being nurtured in another way and on another level.

Look within and see which areas within yourself that you feel would benefit from a healing session or from deep meditation and deep relaxation. Go within the Self and find your inner physician, and see what areas need to be nurtured. As you continue to support the healing process within yourself, you may be able to heal others with a touch, a word, or a thought. Speaking to someone in a conversational, uplifting, inspiring way is helping him or her to heal because you are nurturing. Anytime you can be gracious and speak in positive terms and reaffirm and support someone's hopes and dreams, you are participating in their healing. You become a healer by being an inspirational example to others.

Love

Each person has a different perception, definition, feeling, and thought about love, which may be love of a sport, a game, art, music, life, or the love of a person. Each one of these has a different energy and a different basis upon which it is built. To the different types of

---

[15] Visions are an incredible tool. Here is an exercise you can do quickly, briefly—all you need to do is close yourself off from everything. (However you need to do that: go into a closet, go into a room, go into your car.) Take a moment, do a quick relaxation, and ask: "What do I want to know? What energies are at work that I want to know about?" Your mind will give you a vision, a symbolic picture of the energy at work. Then, with that knowledge in hand, you can focus your intention and approach it with confidence, knowing that you can handle the situation.

love we experience, we attach an emotional component. The love we seek to attain spiritually is Divine Love, which is total acceptance of Self and others. You can only truly love another when you love your Self, not in an egotistical way, but from a place of understanding, knowing that you are a part of the Creative Continuum called God. Through the emotions, mankind is tied into the Material Plane, and it is through the emotions that the dark forces, the negative energies and patternistic behaviors, manifest. This is why you were taught to turn the other cheek and resist not evil[16] because once you begin to resist something, you start feeding it.

The love we experience on a personal, intimate level is more akin to a conceptual approach. For example, in most cases, if you are a woman and you are like your mother, then your significant other will be like your father, based on the unity presented by your parents. If, on the other hand, you and your mother are diametrically opposed, you may choose a man who will continue to stimulate rejection. Each gender seeks to gain the acceptance of Mom, either seeking to emulate her or go the opposite way. Yet when you fall in love, it is more a matter of fulfilling your concepts that relate to the other gender; keep in mind that this also represents an aspect of unity.

As energy, love is an essential cornerstone of a healthy, invigorated life. If you are a guy, then depending upon your relationship with your mother, you will either be just like your dad or the exact opposite. The opposites use rejection as a form of acceptance.

---

[16] "But I say unto you, That ye **resist not** evil: but whosoever shall smite thee on thy right cheek, turn to him the other also.—"Matthew 5:39

Conclusion

There is a Universal Teaching that states, "Every end is a new beginning." You have come to the end of this written material. Within in it you were presented many teachings to help and guide you in ascending to the next level of awareness and consciousness. Some of the material you may have heard or read before. Some concepts and patterns of behavior may be completely new to you. On an intellectual level, you may know some or most of it. However, knowing something and being able to apply is a whole other matter. This is one reason why many self-help programs fail—because they are intellectually based presentations without methods and techniques for application. Their teachings are meant to help, and they often are well-worded and clever, but lack the "how to" so that real and lasting changes can be made.

Having knowledge is one thing. Applying the knowledge is another. It is through the application of that knowledge that wisdom is acquired. When this is achieved, then and only then is true growth accomplished. This information that I have shared with you is akin to scripture found in Luke 24:45: "Then opened He their understanding, that they might understand the scriptures." It is obvious from this statement that Jesus shared with his disciples a perspective of looking at, and understanding, what others could not see, hear, and understand. In fact, here is what is said: "And He said, "Unto you it is given to know the mysteries of the Kingdom of God; but to others in parables, that seeing they might not see, and hearing they might not understand" (Luke 8:10).

This is also why it was reinforced to have eyes that see and ears that hear. Here is what is written: "For this people's heart is waxed gross, and their ears are dull of hearing, and their **eyes** they have closed; lest at any time they should see with their **eyes** and hear with their ears, and should understand with their heart, and should be converted, and I should heal them. But blessed are your **eyes**, for they see: and your ears, for they hear" (Mathew 13:15.(16–

Now is the time for you to become converted to a disciple unto yourself. All of the answers you seek to know and understand are within you. You will be on the path to true enlightenment once you go within and understand the concepts you're working with and how the patterns are showing up in your behaviors. Also important is *knowing* where you are in the cycle that is unfolding and then gaining clarity on what it is you seek to fulfill. Mathew 7:13 has a teaching on this: "Enter ye in at the strait gate [the Self], for wide is the gate, and broad is the way [what man teaches] that leadeth to destruction, and many there be which go in there at. [Just look at the world today.] Because straight is the gate, and narrow is the way [the inward journey], which leadeth unto life [the kingdom is within], **and few** there be that find it."

I can tell you from personal experience that the Universal Teachings, when understood and applied, will bring peace, balance, and harmony into your life on all levels. The Buddha stated, "There are only two mistakes one can make along the road to truth; not going all the way, and not starting. No matter how hard the past you can always begin again. Peace comes from within. Do not seek it without."

•

"Wisdom begins in wonder."
—*Socrates*

"New beginnings are often disguised as painful endings."
—*Lao Tzu*

You have begun your journey by reading and working with this material. Please reach out to me with your experiences, insights, understandings, and accomplishments. Also, if you become "stuck" or want greater clarification or assistance with any aspect of this work, I am here for you at: info@cutateachings.org.

About the Author

Michael Schwartz, N.D. is the Director at the Center for Universal Teachings Applied, a nonprofit organization, where he serves as a wholistic life counselor and naturopathic doctor, specializing in the Mind, Body, Spirit approach. His practice is centered around the spiritual and Universal Teachings presented by the great masters. He is also president of MNP (Michael's® Naturopathic Programs) since 1984. His supplements and health writings can be seen at michaelshealth.com. Michael has worked in the natural food industry since 1976.

Michael is the author of eighteen books, including: *The Universal Teachings Handbook*; *Gospel According to Thomas*; *The Symbolic Interpretation of the Book of Genesis*; *The Symbolic Interpretation of the Book of Exodus*; *The Symbolic Interpretation of the Book of Leviticus*; *Understanding Who You Are and Why You're Here*; *Mind Matters*; *When You Die: How to Master Life and Transition with Personal Power*; *Dream Symbology Dictionary*; *Letting Go*; *The Twelve Disciplines and Spiritual Gifts*; *Laughing on the Outside, Crying on the Inside: Sacrifice Is not the Way to Happiness*; *The Emotional Causes of Diseases*; *Autoimmune Diseases: Why You Have an Immune System*; *Amino Acid Symbology*; *The Seven Causes of Cancer*; *Life Beginnings: Fetal Symbology*; *Naturopathic Healing Handbook*. These books are available at cutateachings.org.

His podcasts can be downloaded at https://michaelsnaturopathytoday.podbean.com

Additional Books from the Author

Purchased these books at <u>cutateachings.org</u>.

BOOKS FOR THE SPIRIT

The Universal Teachings Handbook
This book comprises a body of knowledge and a common ground of all the religions and philosophies of the great teachers in history—Lao Tzu, Buddha, Jesus, Ra, Krishna, and others. Regardless of your faith, life path, or practice, the Universal Principles and the Universal Teachings are applicable to your life because they transcend all boundaries. The Teachings will help you to understand how your life works at the deepest subconscious level. As you incorporate the understandings and applications of the Teachings into your life, you will begin to see change and growth almost immediately. They offer a way to gain control over emotions, become at peace with your life, and look at life and relationships from a position of strength and greater personal power. The Teachings will provide a foundation for living, thinking and experiencing life, helping you to see and understand the deeper intricacies and the hidden energies at work in everything you experience.

The Gospel According to Thomas: A Symbolic Interpretation
This book is an examination of the sayings and Teachings of Jesus as expressed in the Gospel According to Thomas, one of many scrolls found in Nag Hammadi, Egypt, in 1943. The scrolls are considered authentic, and this one appears to have been written while Jesus was alive whereas the New Testament Gospels were written seven decades after his death. In fact, many biblical scholars believe these Teachings are the foundation of those echoed in the gospels of the New Testament. These 114 Teachings, when applied, lead to a masterful spiritual life. Mastery is the result of emotional control based on understandings and insights achieved through the application of the Teachings presented. The Universal Teachings are based on the Immutable Laws of God and therefore are applicable to every person, regardless of their religious perspective or conviction.

The Symbolic Interpretation of the Book of Genesis
The Symbolic Interpretation of the Book of Exodus
The Symbolic Interpretation of the Book of Leviticus
Each book offered is a symbolic interpretation of what is said in each book of the Bible. This is done by line, paragraph, or event in each chapter.

BOOKS FOR THE MIND

Mind Matters
This book lights the path to understanding how your conscious and your subconscious influence, and even determine, how you feel and what you do every day. *Mind Matters* teaches you how to realign your mental software. By using symbology, tapping into the God force, and blending spirituality with material reality, you can become your true self, living out your divine nature, rather than who you were programmed to be.

Letting Go
This book is a guide to understanding what is essential to know in order to let go. You cannot let go until you understand why you are still holding on. This book explores the emotional connections to cancer, arthritis, diabetes, weight issues, and relationships, which the hardest situations to let go of. This work contains methods and techniques for understanding why you are holding on. With this key information, it becomes easier to finally let go and move forward in your life with great health and in good spirits—and you can stop your personal history from repeating itself.

When You Die: How to Master Life and Transition with Personal Power
This work details what you can do now to live a meaningful life filled with self-knowledge. Additionally, this book explores what takes place on the other side of this dimension where the recently deceased go. Some walk, and some run with joy; others drag their feet out of fear of what is on the other side of the doorway called death. This perspective will show what takes place and why.

Laughing on the Outside, Crying on the Inside: Sacrifice Is not the Way to Happiness
This book explores the concept of sacrifice and how it affects the lives of those involved. Sacrifice, like everything, can be good or bad. It can lead to many problems. Understanding the energies involved gives you the opportunity to change both the situation and the outcome.

Understanding Who You Are and Why You're Here
This book is about life and its true purpose which is mastering the material plane, the dimension we live in, and reuniting with the God Force, the Creative Continuum. Within these pages you will learn why we are here and what we are here to accomplish. Yes, there really is a purpose to life beyond self-gratification.

The Dream Symbology Dictionary
With this comprehensive compendium of symbols that appear in dreams, visions, and in day-to-day experiences, readers discover through detailed definitions that dreams have the potential to change their lives. With simple, fascinating guidelines to dream interpretation, the enigmatic misadventures of your sleeping mind provide clues for profound insights. Dreams are jewels in the rough that have the potential to change your life. This book also provides techniques for recalling dreams. Dreams are an essential part of the guidance system the mind uses to inform you of concepts you are working with, their patterns of behavior, and where you are in the flow

of them. Dreams are retrocognitive and precognitive. They are also based on the Universal Teaching: "We look back in order to see ahead."

The Twelve Disciplines and Spiritual Gifts

Each of the 12 disciples of Jesus can be seen to represent or be symbolic of a spiritual gift we possess. The Bible itself is a handbook for spiritual growth and development, leading to higher consciousness. The benefit of a discipline is that it will help you achieve your goals. In terms of goals, there are four different goals, since there are four aspects of the self. This book shows you how adopting each of the twelve disciplines will help you accomplish your goals.

BOOKS FOR THE BODY

Life Beginnings: Fetal Symbology

This book is an examination of fetal development. As the fetus develops within the womb, physical systems, glands, organs, and functions unfold in a particular process at very specific times. I have examined those times and coincided them with the numerology I use based on the Universal Teachings so that each developmental stage and its numerical significance gives one a tremendous insight as to the energies at work—not only in the developing fetus but in life itself.

Amino Acid Symbology

This book is an examination of the amino acids that create our DNA and proteins, which are the foundation of the functioning of the body. Each amino acid and its symbolic or energetic significance is viewed in terms of what it does within the body and what it represents on an emotional level. When this is understood, one can see the role that understanding plays in the development of one's life and health.

Autoimmune Diseases: Why You Have an Immune System!

This book examines over seventy of the common autoimmune diseases. The major difference between this and all other books written about autoimmune diseases is that I disagree with the current medical thinking. I believe the body is doing exactly what it is supposed to do. It is seeking to eliminate cells that do not belong in the body. Each area of the body under attack is doing so to help guide you to a deep-seated concept in your subconscious mind. By understanding the true cause of dis-ease, you can then begin to eliminate the condition from your life.

The Seven Causes of Cancer: How to Prevent and Eliminate Them

This work shows you the seven causes of cancer and what you can do to prevent, eliminate, and control the growth of this disease. Each cause has a specific source of origination. Knowing what they are provides you with the insights as to what you can do to live a great life free of cancer. If you are dealing with cancer, this will show you why and what to do about it.

The Naturopathic Healing Handbook

This is a definitive reference for natural healing—essential guide to understanding how to live a healthy life. All of the work in here can also be found in the *Disease Symbology Handbook* with the emotional understandings for each condition.

The Emotional Causes of Diseases
A reference work for true healing, this book is the definitive guide to how emotions are the real causes of disease, common physical conditions, and states of mind. It's an almanac of Universal Guiding Principles expressed as Universal Teachings and keys to the healing properties of the mind, nutrients, herbs and supplements are presented. You'll uncover a powerful system for healing and recovery in all aspects of life—health, financial, social, and psychological—by using inspired Teachings to reveal the root causes of physical and emotional disharmony.

www.ingramcontent.com/pod-product-compliance
Lightning Source LLC
Chambersburg PA
CBHW052112020426
42335CB00021B/2727